BASIC
HAND
SPLINTING
A Pattern-
Designing
Approach

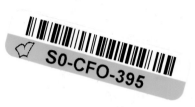
SO-CFO-395

BASIC HAND SPLINTING
A Pattern-Designing Approach

Judith Hunt Kiel, M.S., O.T.R.

*Assistant Professor and Curriculum Coordinator, Occupational Therapy
Program, Division of Allied Health Sciences, Indiana University
School of Medicine, Indianapolis*

Illustrated by

Catherine Erickson Barrett, M.S., O.T.R.

*Director of Therapeutic Activities, Hooverwood, Indianapolis Jewish
Home for the Aged; Adjunct Associate Professor, Occupational Therapy
Program, Division of Allied Health Sciences, Indiana University
School of Medicine, Indianapolis*

Susie Young Baxter, B.F.A.

Freelance Artist, Indianapolis

Little, Brown and Company, Boston/Toronto

Copyright © 1983 by Judith Hunt Kiel

First Edition

Third Printing

All rights reserved. No part of this book may be reproduced in any form or by any electronic or mechanical means, including information storage and retrieval systems, without permission in writing from the publisher, except by a reviewer who may quote brief passages in a review.

Library of Congress Catalog Card No. 82-83349

ISBN 0-316-49177-2

Printed in the United States of America

KP

For my students:

The former ones who taught me so much,
the current ones who continue to challenge me, and
the future ones who will guide me to new horizons.

Contents

Preface

In my teaching of splinting I have found that students appreciate concrete information that can be used to understand the principles of splinting. With this kind of specific information as a foundation, those who have pursued the study and practice of hand rehabilitation have learned other methods easily, but, even more importantly, have developed their own methods based on sound data.

It is for students, as well as for therapists who have not pursued hand rehabilitation but have an occasional need for a basic splinting reference, that this book has been written. In addition to a clear explanation of the principles of splinting theory, a detailed explanation of how to make a pattern for a splint is also presented. With this information a therapist should be able to use the information given as well as adapt it to the design of other splints.

I wish to express my appreciation to all the people who have encouraged and inspired me while working on this project. Without the initial work and enthusiasm of T. Kay Carl I would not have developed an interest in splinting. The prodding guidance, excellent critique, and constant encouragement of Shereen D. Farber were invaluable.

Grateful acknowledgment is due several people who read various chapters and offered excellent suggestions. These people include Lucinda Dale, Chris Kozal, Michelle Landers, Chris Paulik, Barb Pfoser, and Paula Walt who, as students, were capable of accurately assessing whether this material might be appreciated by other students.

I want to thank the Occupational Therapy Department at the James Whitcomb Riley Hospital for Children, Indiana University Medical Center, Indianapolis and the Occupational Therapy Department at St. Francis Hospital Center, Beech Grove, Indiana for permission to use their forms for exercises and splint care.

I feel deep appreciation for my husband, Gregory A. Kiel, for his patience, support, and suggestions. The entire book is greatly enhanced by the illustrations provided by Catherine E. Barrett and Susie Young Baxter. In addition I owe thanks to Sue Ward, whose typing skills were used to their fullest.

Finally, I wish to thank Barbara O. Ward, Little, Brown Allied Health Editor, who was a great source of support and knowledge; and Priscilla Hurdle, Little, Brown Book Editor, who did an excellent job of ensuring that this text made sense.

J.H.K.

BASIC HAND SPLINTING
A Pattern-Designing Approach

1. Anatomy of the Hand

It is important for a therapist engaged in splinting the hand to have a thorough knowledge of the anatomy and kinesiology of the part being splinted. This text will briefly cover the kind of information required in the clinic while splinting the hand, that is sometimes not easily found in anatomy and hand rehabilitation books. The topics covered include

A. Terms essential to splinting

    1. Bones of the hand and forearm
    2. Joints of the hand
    3. Surface anatomy
    4. Soft tissue

B. Intrinsic muscles

    1. Definition
    2. List of the muscles
    3. Origin and insertion
    4. Innervation of the muscles
    5. Primary and secondary actions of the muscles

C. Extrinsic Muscles

    1. Definition
    2. List of the muscles
    3. Origin and insertion
    4. Innervation of the muscles
    5. Primary and secondary actions of the muscles

D. Normal hand function

    1. Volar hand creases
    2. Functional position
    3. Arches of the hand
    4. Dual obliquity
    5. Prehension patterns
    6. Patient education

E. Classic appearance of some common hand injuries

    1. Radial nerve severance
    2. Median nerve severance
    3. Ulnar nerve severance
    4. Median/ulnar nerve severance
    5. Rheumatoid arthritis
    6. Burn

At the conclusion of this chapter a list of references is suggested for further study of hand anatomy and rehabilitation.

Terms Essential to Splinting

In defining anatomical terms, some are best understood through illustration, for example, the names of the bones in the hand in Figure 1-1, and the names of the joints in the hand in Figure 1-2.

Other terms that must be defined are the *dorsal surface* of the hand, the back of the hand where the knuckles are located. The *volar* or *palmar surface* of the hand is the concave part, on the side of the finger pads. The *radial side* of the hand is the side where the thumb is located. The side of the hand with the little finger is called the *ulnar side*. The lateral side of the hand always indicates the radial side. This is clear when the hand is viewed with the body in the anatomical position. Other terms that must be understood in any discussion of splinting of the hand include *distal*, farthest from the point of attachment, and *proximal*, nearest to the point of attachment.

The terminology used for the fingers varies. Sometimes the fingers are

Figure 1-1. Bones of the hand and forearm.

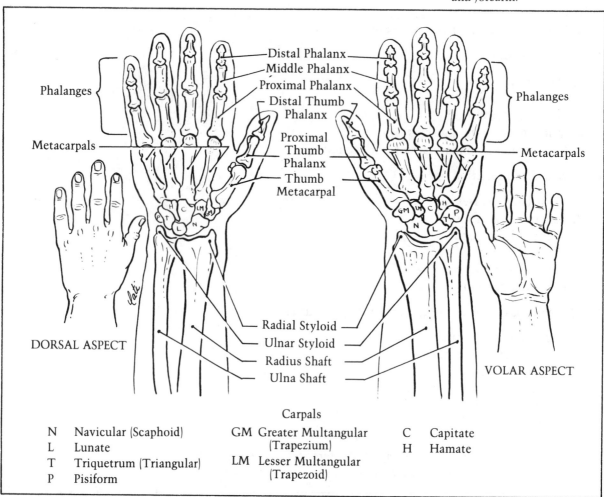

N	Navicular (Scaphoid)	GM Greater Multangular (Trapezium)	C Capitate
L	Lunate	LM Lesser Multangular (Trapezoid)	H Hamate
T	Triquetrum (Triangular)		
P	Pisiform		

referred to as *digits* and are numbered from one to five, with the thumb designated number one and the small finger number five. Other sources name the thumb but number the other fingers one through four. In order to avoid confusion, others name all the fingers: thumb, index, middle or long, ring, and little or small. Numbering the fingers is more common when designating a specific joint or bone. This text uses the naming system when mention is made of the entire finger, but also uses the number system from one to five when discussing specific bones and joints for making splinting patterns.

The joints of the hand and fingers are encapsulated by the muscles and tendons of the hand, as well as the palmar aponeurosis, the flexor retinaculum, the extensor hoods, and the flexor tendon sheaths. The joints of the hand are prone to adhesions and stiffness following immobilization for even a short period of time, because of the hand's complex anatomy. Another danger is edema in the hand caused by disease, injury, or lack of circulation, occasionally caused by a tight splint. Because the tissues in the hand are so tightly packed that there is no extra room for any foreign substance, edema that is not eliminated rapidly can cause serious, and possibly irreparable, damage to the normal function of the hand.

Figure 1-2. Joints of the hand and wrist.

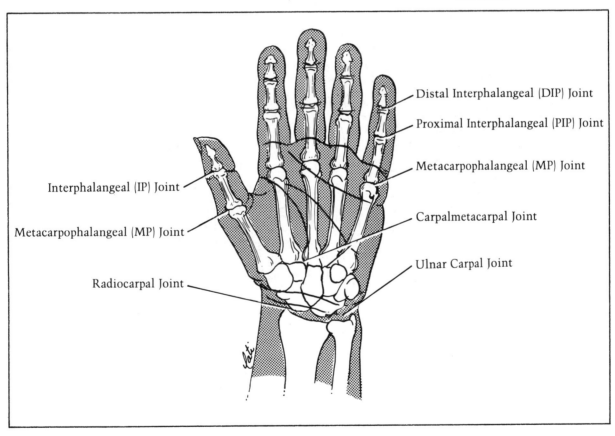

Distal Interphalangeal (DIP) Joint

Proximal Interphalangeal (PIP) Joint

Metacarpophalangeal (MP) Joint

Carpalmetacarpal Joint

Ulnar Carpal Joint

Interphalangeal (IP) Joint

Metacarpophalangeal (MP) Joint

Radiocarpal Joint

Intrinsic and Extrinsic Muscles

Intrinsic muscles (Table 1, Fig. 1–3 and 1–4) are those that are located entirely distal to the wrist. The tendons of extrinsic muscles (Table 2) cross the carpal area into the palm and fingers, but the muscle belly is located in the forearm. Some extrinsic muscles also cross the elbow joint.

An extrinsic muscle has varying degrees of effect on all of the joints that it crosses. An example of this is the flexor digitorum profundus, which originates on the anterior surface of the ulna and inserts at the bases of the distal phalanges of the second through fifth digits. The primary action of this muscle is flexion of the distal interphalangeal joints, but it also assists with the flexion of the proximal interphalangeal joints, the metacarpal phalangeal joints, and the wrist.

There are three nerves providing innervation to the hand. The specific muscles that they innervate are found in Tables 1 and 2. A picture of the sensory innervation pattern is found in Figure 1–5.

Figure 1-3. Deep intrinsic muscles.

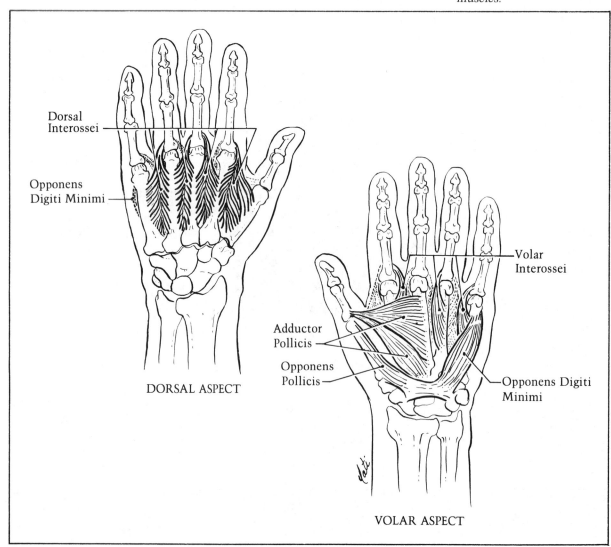

Dorsal Interossei

Opponens Digiti Minimi

DORSAL ASPECT

Volar Interossei

Adductor Pollicis

Opponens Pollicis

Opponens Digiti Minimi

VOLAR ASPECT

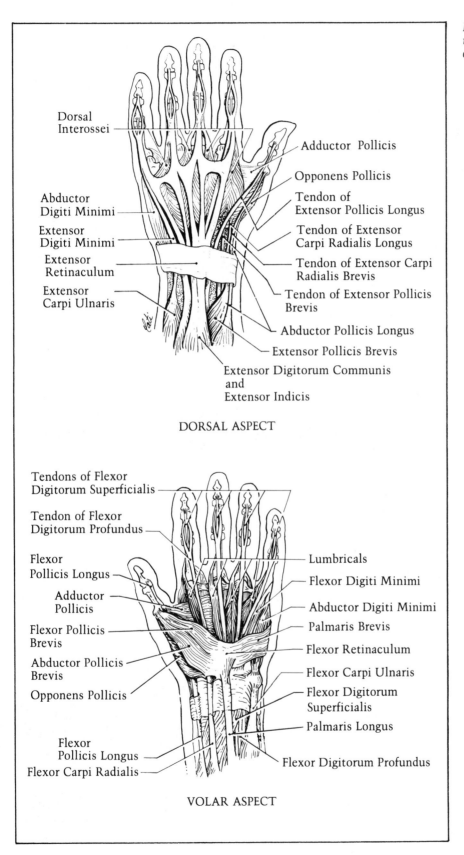

Figure 1-4. Superficial intrinsic muscles and tendons of extrinsic muscles.

Dorsal Interossei

Adductor Pollicis

Opponens Pollicis

Tendon of Extensor Pollicis Longus

Abductor Digiti Minimi

Tendon of Extensor Carpi Radialis Longus

Extensor Digiti Minimi

Tendon of Extensor Carpi Radialis Brevis

Extensor Retinaculum

Tendon of Extensor Pollicis Brevis

Extensor Carpi Ulnaris

Abductor Pollicis Longus

Extensor Pollicis Brevis

Extensor Digitorum Communis and Extensor Indicis

DORSAL ASPECT

Tendons of Flexor Digitorum Superficialis

Tendon of Flexor Digitorum Profundus

Flexor Pollicis Longus

Lumbricals

Flexor Digiti Minimi

Adductor Pollicis

Abductor Digiti Minimi

Flexor Pollicis Brevis

Palmaris Brevis

Flexor Retinaculum

Abductor Pollicis Brevis

Flexor Carpi Ulnaris

Opponens Pollicis

Flexor Digitorum Superficialis

Palmaris Longus

Flexor Pollicis Longus

Flexor Carpi Radialis

Flexor Digitorum Profundus

VOLAR ASPECT

Table 1. *Intrinsic Muscles* [1, 4, 6, 7, 8, 9, 11]

Muscles	Origin	Insertion	Innervation	Primary action	Secondary action
Abductor pollicis brevis	Radial border of the flexor retinaculum, navicular, and ridge of greater multangular	Radial side of base of proximal phalanx and extensor mechanism	Median	Abduction of thumb at right angle to index finger; Opposition of thumb to all fingers; Stabilization of thumb	Extension of interphalangeal joint of thumb
Flexor pollicis brevis	Superficial head: flexor retinaculum and ridge of greater multangular; Deep head: lesser multangular and capitate	Base of proximal phalanx and extensor mechanism	Superficial head: median; Deep head: ulnar	Adduction of 1st metacarpal bone; Flexion of 1st metacarpal phalangeal joint	Extension of interphalangeal joint of thumb
Opponens pollicis	Flexor retinaculum and ridge of greater multangular	Entire length of radial border of first metacarpal	Median	Flexion and rotation of 1st metacarpal bone toward palmar surface of second, third, fourth, and fifth fingers	None
Adductor pollicis	Oblique head: capitate, lesser multangular, bases of second and third metacarpal bones, and palmar ligaments; Transverse head: palmar surface of third metacarpal	Ulnar side of base of proximal phalanx of thumb and extensor mechanism	Ulnar	Adduction of thumb from abduction; Assistance with opposition; Flexion of metacarpal phalangeal joint of thumb	Extension of interphalangeal joint of thumb
Abductor digiti minimi (quinti)	Pisiform, pisohamate ligament, and tendon of flexor carpi ulnaris	Medial border of proximal phalanx of little finger and extensor mechanism	Ulnar	Abduction of little finger; Stabilization of fifth metacarpal phalangeal joint in opposition	Extension of both interphalangeal joints of little finger
Flexor digiti minimi (quinti brevis)	Hook of the hamate and flexor retinaculum	Base of proximal phalanx of little finger, volar to insertion of abductor	Ulnar	Flexion of fifth metacarpal phalangeal joint	Flexion and adduction of fifth metacarpal bone
Opponens digiti minimi (quinti)	Hook of the hamate and flexor retinaculum	Entire length of ulnar border of fifth metacarpal bone	Ulnar	Flexion and rotation of fifth metacarpal bone toward thumb in opposition	Stabilization of fifth metacarpal bone
Dorsal interossei (4)	Each has 2 origins from adjacent metacarpal heads	Proximal phalanx of finger it moves	Ulnar	Abduction of index, middle, and ring fingers from the midline	Assistance of lumbricals with flexion of metacarpal phalangeal joints and extension of interphalangeal joints
Volar interossei (3)	Each has single origin from second, fourth, or fifth metacarpal bone	Respectively, second, fourth, or fifth proximal phalanx	Ulnar	Adduction of second, fourth, or fifth finger toward middle finger	Assistance of lumbricals with flexion of metacarpal phalangeal joints and extension of interphalangeal joints
Lumbricals (4)	Each has own origin from respective tendons of flexor digitorum profundus	With dorsal interossei into respective bases of proximal phalanges	Radial two: median; Ulnar two: ulnar	Flexion of metacarpal phalangeal joints and extension of interphalangeal joints; Coordinates fine movement of metacarpal, phalangeal, and interphalangeal joints	Assistance with rotation of index finger; Stabilization of interphalangeal joints in extension
Palmaris brevis	Ulnar side of transverse carpal ligament and palmar aponeurosis	Skin on ulner border of hand	Ulnar	Deepens hollow of hand	Corrugation of skin on ulnar side of palm

Table 2. Extrinsic Muscles [1, 4, 6, 7, 8, 9, 11]

Muscles	Origin	Insertion	Innervation	Primary action	Secondary action
Flexor pollicis longus	Anterior surface of radius	Base of distal phalanx of thumb	Median	Flexion of interphalangeal joint of thumb	Wrist flexion; Thumb adduction
Extensor pollicis longus	Radial border of posterior aspect of ulna	Radial aspect of distal phalanx of thumb	Radial	Extension of interphalangeal joint of thumb; External rotation of thumb	Wrist extension; Radial abduction of thumb; Thumb adduction
Extensor pollicis brevis	Ulnar border of posterior surface of radius	Base of proximal phalanx of thumb	Radial	Extension and stabilization of first metacarpal phalangeal joint	None
Abductor pollicis longus	Posterior aspect of radius, interosseous membrane, slip on posterior aspect of ulna	Base of first metacarpal bone	Radial	Stabilization of thumb during activity of extensors; Abduction of thumb radially	None
Flexor digitorum profundus	Anterior surface of ulna, interosseous membrane, deep fascia of forearm	Base of distal phalanges of second-fifth fingers on palmar surface	Radial two: median; Ulnar two: ulnar	Flexion of second-fifth distal interphalangeal joints	Assistance with wrist, metacarpal phalangeal, and proximal interphalangeal flexion
Flexor digitorum superficialis (sublimus)	Medial epicondyle of humerus, coronoid process of ulna, ulnar collateral ligament, and outer border of radius	Bases of middle phalanges of second-fifth fingers	Median	Flexion of second-fifth proximal interphalangeal joints	Assistance with wrist and metacarpal phalangeal flexion
Extensor digitorum communis (extensor digitorum, extensor communis)	Lateral epicondyle of humerus	Composes extensor expansion on dorsal surface of middle and distal phalanges second-fifth fingers	Radial	Extension of metacarpal phalangeal joints of second-fifth fingers; Extension of proximal and distal interphalangeal joints of second-fifth fingers when metacarpal phalangeal joints are stabilized	Abduction of fingers when in extension; Assistance with wrist extension; Assistance with elbow flexion; Stabilization of hand for finger flexion
Extensor indicis (indicis proprius)	Radial border of posterior surface of ulna	Tendon to index finger from extensor digitorum communis	Radial	Extension of metacarpal phalangeal joints of index finger	None
Extensor digiti minimi	Lateral epicondyle of humerus	Extension expansion of little finger	Radial	Extension of metacarpal phalangeal joint of little finger	None
Flexor carpi radialis	Medial epicondyle of humerus	Bases of the second and third metacarpal bones	Median	Flexion of wrist	Assistance with radial deviation of wrist
Flexor carpi ulnaris	One head: medial epicondyle of humerus; Second head: posterior border of ulna	Pisiform and base of fifth metacarpal bone	Ulnar	Flexion of wrist	Assistance with ulnar deviation of wrist
Extensor carpi radialis longus	Lateral epicondylar ridge of humerus and lateral intermuscular septum	Dorsal surface of base of the second metacarpal bone	Radial	Extension of wrist	Assistance with radial deviation of wrist
Extensor carpi radialis brevis	Lateral epicondyle of humerus	Base of third metacarpal bone	Radial	Extension of wrist	Assistance with radial deviation of wrist
Extensor carpi ulnaris	Lateral epicondyle of humerus and posterior border of ulna	Base of fifth metacarpal bone	Radial	Extension of wrist	Assistance with ulnar deviation of wrist
Palmaris longus	Medial epicondyle of humerus	Flexor retinaculum and palmar aponeurosis	Median	Tightening of palmar fascia	Assistance with flexion of wrist

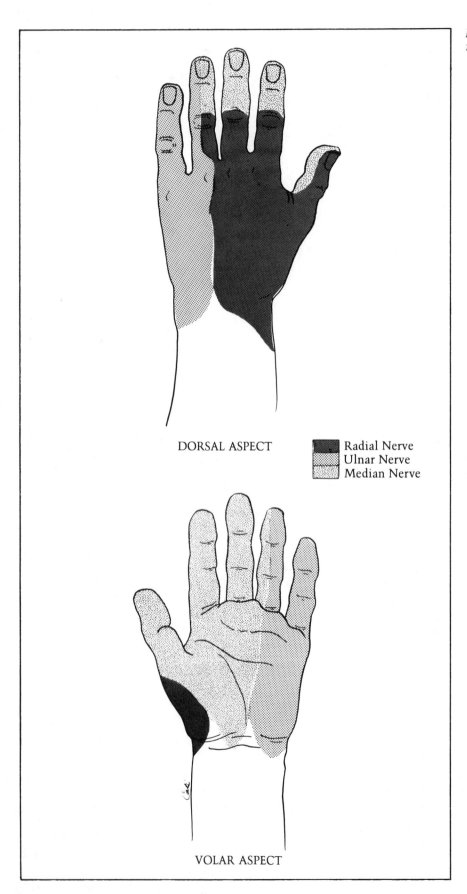

DORSAL ASPECT

■ Radial Nerve
Ulnar Nerve
Median Nerve

VOLAR ASPECT

Figure 1-5. Pattern of sensory innervation.

Normal Hand Function

With the large number of bones in the hand, there are obviously a large number of joints where these bones articulate. The mobility without pain of all of these joints is essential for the hand to function in all of its intricate capacities. Any splint that is applied must allow as much motion as possible, considering that the diagnosis requires the use of a splint. Using a splint that immobilizes any joint requires good reason for this immobilization, and if medically acceptable, exercises must be done regularly to maintain strength and range of motion.

When the joints are mobile, the soft tissue surrounding the bone (skin, connective tissue, and superficial and deep fascia) must give and adjust. These adjustments are the creases where the skin on that particular hand has chosen to bend as the hand performs its work. These creases (Fig. 1–6), although very near the bony joint, are not necessarily directly on top of them. Because the creases are in soft tissue, they also tend to move slightly as the joint goes through its range of motion (Fig. 1–7).

If a joint is to be allowed movement with a splint in place, this splint must not cross either the bony joint or the crease caused by that joint. The end or edge of a splint must be just short of the bony joint and the crease at that joint. If no motion is to be permitted in the joint, the splint should completely cover the joint and continue to the next joint, where the same principles apply.

One major goal of occupational therapy is to help people function as independently as possible. When splinting, remember this goal, and maintain the splinted hand in the functional position at all times. Whenever possible, the patient should be able to perform normal tasks with the splint in place. (This depends on the type of splint used and its purpose. Some splints deliberately eliminate all function.) Even if the patient cannot perform every task

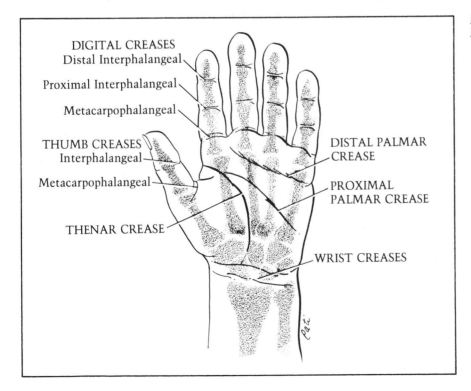

Figure 1-6. Relationship of hand creases to bony joints.

DIGITAL CREASES
Distal Interphalangeal
Proximal Interphalangeal
Metacarpophalangeal

THUMB CREASES
Interphalangeal
Metacarpophalangeal

THENAR CREASE

DISTAL PALMAR CREASE

PROXIMAL PALMAR CREASE

WRIST CREASES

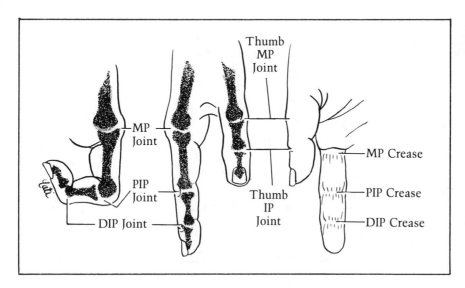

Figure 1-7. The relationship of hand creases to bony joints changes with motion.

with the splint on, the use of the functional position helps ensure the ability to perform normally after the splint is removed. A splint that does not place the hand in a functional position may destroy what otherwise might have been normal performance. See Figure 1–8 for an illustration of what Wynn Parry [11] has described as the functional position for the joints of the upper extremity.

Remember that the functional position for a particular patient may differ slightly from the position described by Wynn Parry because of heredity, habit, or occupational requirements. For this reason, each patient must be evaluated for the best position of function prior to splinting the hand. Individual variations can be determined by examination and interview. It is important to look at the patient's "normal" hand as a reference. The physician may request that the patient be splinted in a slightly different position, and

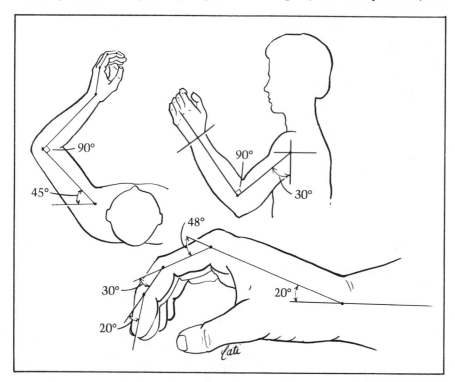

Figure 1-8. Functional position of the upper extremity. Wrist: 20-degree extension (dorsiflexion); metacarpal phalangeal joints: 45-degree flexion; proximal interphalangeal joints: 30-degree flexion; distal interphalangeal joints: 20-degree flexion; thumb placed in half palmar abduction and half opposition with its interphalangeal joint in slight flexion; elbow: 90-degree flexion in midprone position; shoulder: 45-degree abduction, 30-degree flexion, and neutral position.

those instructions must also be considered. Communication and discussion with the physician about the final splinted position is essential.

As seen in the views of the functional position (Fig. 1–8), the hand is not flat. There are arches that must be maintained in order to achieve the position of function. One of these is the transverse metacarpal arch (Fig. 1–9). Examination of the cross section of the metacarpal heads in a functional position indicates that the third metacarpal is more dorsal than the rest of the metacarpals. The second and fourth metacarpals rest slightly volar to the third, but at approximately the same height as one another. The fifth metacarpal head is the most volar of these four metacarpals. The thumb (first metacarpal) is more mobile than the others, and therefore rests in a variety of positions. The first metacarpal head, however, should be either directly volar to the second metacarpal head, or volar and slightly radial to the second metacarpal head. It usually lies more volar than the fifth metacarpal head. During activity this arch deepens and the great mobility of the first, fourth, and fifth metacarpals becomes evident. When splinting, it is important to maintain the transverse metacarpal arch in at least a functional position. It is even better if room can be allowed for excursion beyond just that position (assuming that the splint is designed to allow motion).

Figure 1-9. Transverse metacarpal arch (after Netter).

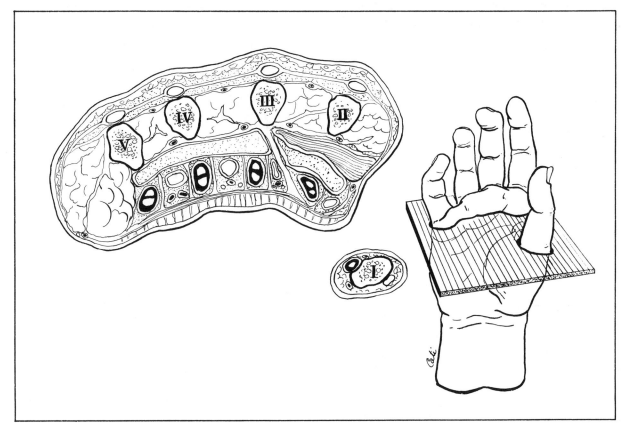

The longitudinal arch (Fig. 1–10) is what permits the metacarpophalangeal (MP), proximal interphalangeal (PIP), and distal interphalangeal (DIP) joints to flex. Any splint covering these joints should have some curvature in these areas (as seen in the functional position) to prevent the finger joints from stiffening in a straight position.

The proximal transverse arch (carpal arch) is formed by the carpal bones and is held in place by the flexor retinaculum. This ligament, in combination with the carpal bones, makes up the carpal tunnel. Several of the extrinsic muscle tendons, along with the median nerve, pass through this tunnel. The carpal tunnel serves as a fulcrum for the wrist flexors and provides their mechanical advantage. The carpal arch is not mobile and does not usually require extra consideration for support.

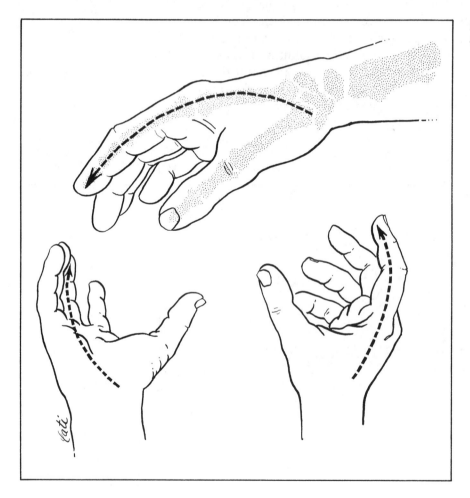

Figure 1-10. Longitudinal arch.

Owing to the arches of the hand and the different lengths of the metacarpals, objects are held in the hand in two oblique angles. Because the metacarpals are longer on the radial side of the hand, an object held in the hand forms an angle oblique to the bones of the forearm (radius and ulna). The object in the hand will be more distal to the elbow on the radial side than on the unlar side, and approximately parallel to the heads of the metacarpals. Figure 1–11 indicates by the rod in the hand the approximate angle of obliquity normally seen in the hand.

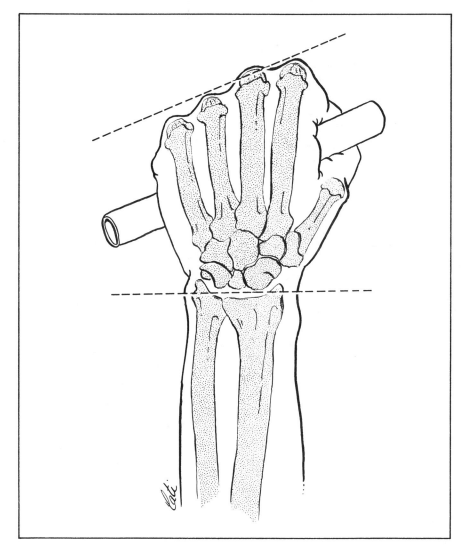

Figure 1-11. Oblique angle of objects held in hand caused by the differing lengths of the metacarpals.

The second oblique angle will show the object placed dorsally (or higher) on the radial side than on the ulnar side. The object is not parallel to the floor when the hand is pronated. This angle is indicated by the rod in the hand in Figure 1-12. This angle is caused by the transverse metacarpal arch and the mobility of the fourth and fifth metacarpals when the hand is being used.

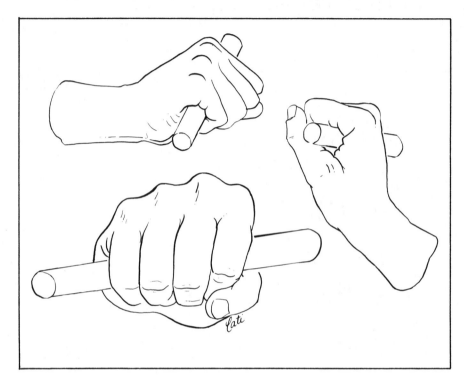

Figure 1-12. Oblique angle of objects held in hand caused by the transverse metacarpal arch.

In order for a splint to fit correctly these two angles must be respected. The radial side of the splint must be more distal than the ulnar side [1], and the splint must be higher on the radial side than the ulnar side. Figure 1–13 shows the two oblique angles as they should be seen in a splint.

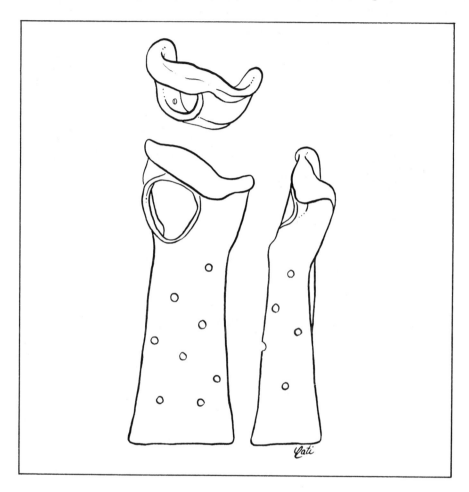

Figure 1-13. Dual obliquity in a splint.

In normal use the hand assumes many positions requiring varying degrees of precision and strength. Every normal hand has the capacity for assuming the same positions, or prehension patterns. There are six general prehension patterns, three of which focus mainly on precision activities. These patterns for precision are called *pinch* (Figs. 1–14 A, B, C). Pinch is used in handling small objects that are held between the tips of the thumb and one or more fingers [6]. The other three prehension patterns, called *grasp*, focus mainly on strength. Grasp is used in handling large objects and uses the thumb and all four fingers holding the object against the palm (Figs. 1–15 A, B, C).

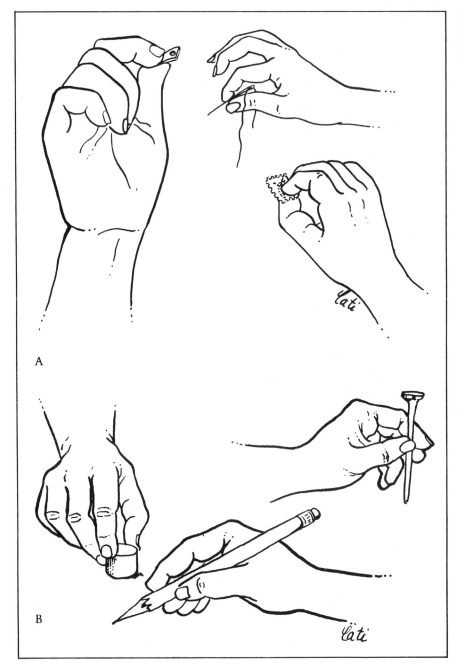

Figure 1-14. Three types of pinch. A. Tip prehension. B. Palmar prehension (three-jaw chuck).

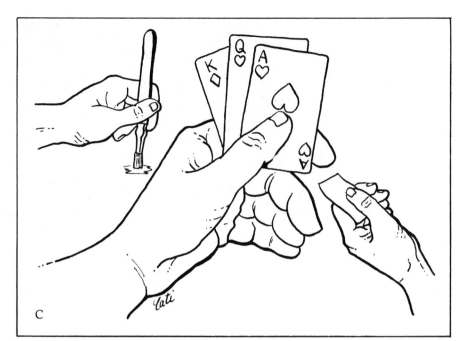

Figure 1-14C. Lateral prehension.

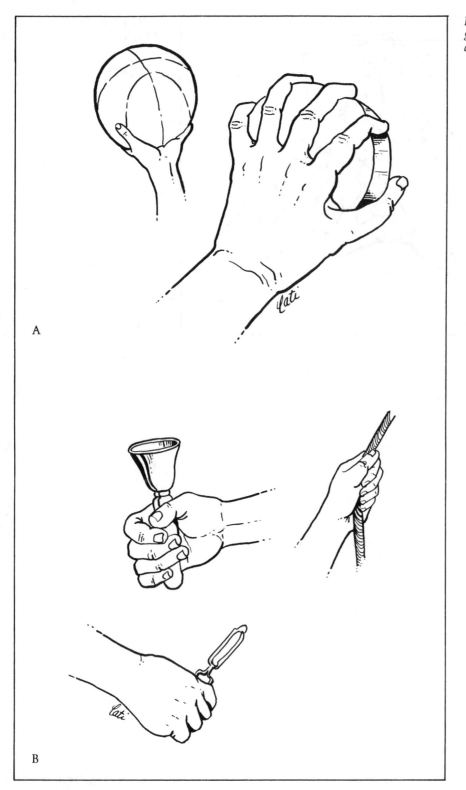

Figure 1-15. Three types of grasp. A. Gross grasp. B. Cylindrical grasp.

A

B

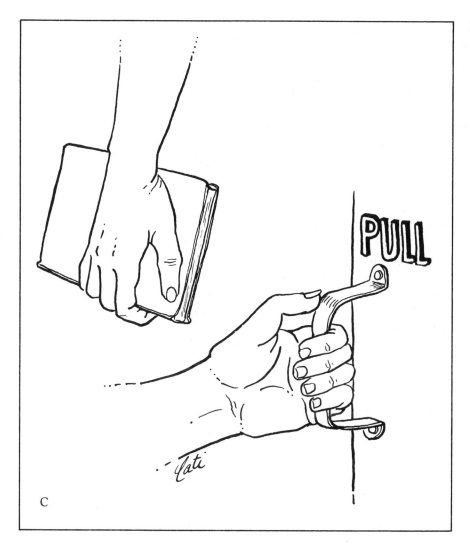

C

Figure 1-15C. Hook grasp.

Notice in the illustrations that all of these prehension patterns have some common characteristics. These include wrist extension, some degree of finger flexion, and thumb opposition.

When making splints, it is important that the splint permits as many of the prehension patterns as possible. This directly depends, of course, on the type of splint being used, as the purpose of some splints is to rest the entire hand or a particular joint. If this is the case, then one, some, or all of the prehension patterns will be eliminated. However, when the splint is removed all of the prehension patterns should be restored. One of the reasons for allowing function of as many prehension patterns as possible is to maintain maximum mobility in the joints (see p. 3). A second reason is to increase the likelihood of patient acceptance. Ideally, when a splint is given to someone to wear, its benefit will be immediately evident. If this benefit is not immediate or obvious, the therapist must be able to explain why it is not, and why it is definitely worth the patient's effort to continue treatment. The therapist should also be able to describe what improvement will be like and how the person can recognize its earliest signs. If the above procedure is not followed, it is unlikely that the splint will be worn, because the patient will see no purpose in going through the inconvenience [2, 3].

Patient Education

Knowledge of anatomy is important to the therapist in hand rehabilitation in order to plan proper treatment. It is also necessary to explain anatomical basics to the patient because, the therapist can lay out a course, but it is the patient who must direct efforts so that maximal improvement will ensue. The patient's comprehension of the extent of injury to the structures and the value of the diverse therapy routines is fundamental to the treatment [5]. The therapist is usually the one to explain the details, because the patient thinks of questions during therapy rather than when the doctor is present.

Classic Appearance of Some Common Hand Injuries

Figures 1–16 through 1–21 show the classic appearance of some of the more common hand injuries before treatment. The purpose of these illustrations is to give the beginner an indication of what a patient's problem might be. Discussion of each patient's specific problem with the physician is essential prior to the initiation of treatment. Also, further research into specific muscle, tendon, ligament, nerve, and soft tissue involvement is urged before treatment. Note in these illustrations the flattened arches and misshapen

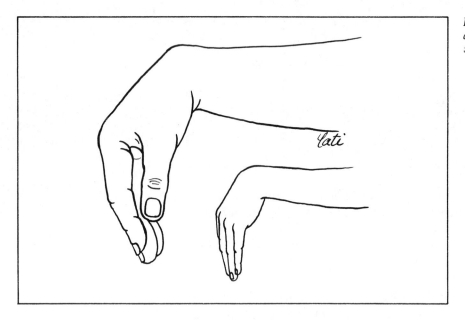

Figure 1-16. Classic appearance of radial nerve severance—wrist drop.

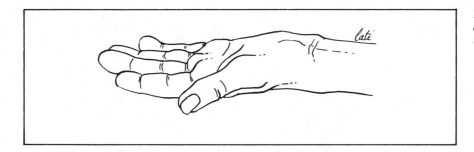

Figure 1-17. Classic appearance of median nerve severance—ape hand.

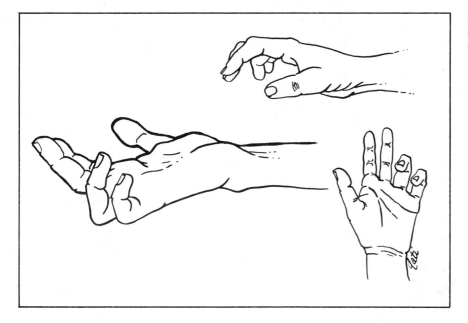

Figure 1-18. Classic appearance of ulnar nerve severance—claw hand.

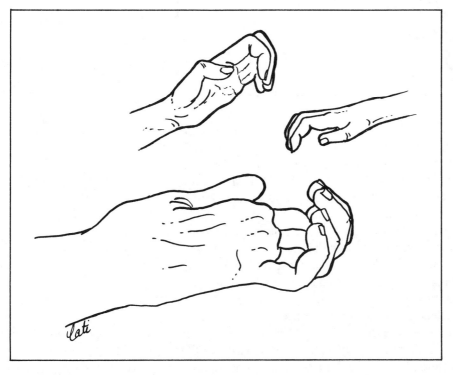

Figure 1-19. Classic appearance of median/ulnar nerve severance.

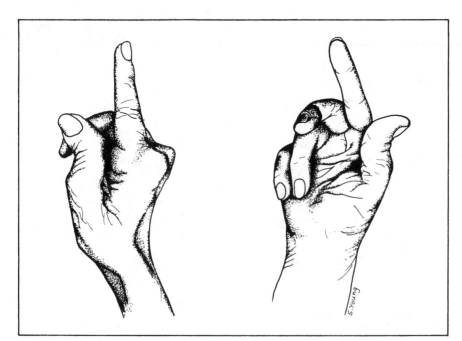

Figure 1-20. Classic appearance of arthritic hand.

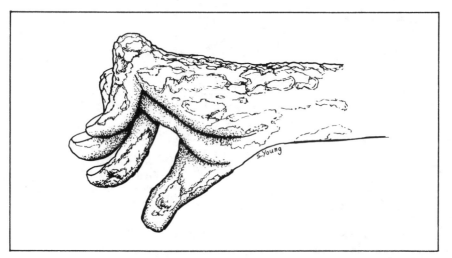

Figure 1-21. Classic appearance of burned hand.

fingers, joints, and/or soft tissue, as these all affect the fitting of a splint. Note also that in the case of a burned hand the physician may ask for a splinted position that deviates from the traditional functional position. The position requested is sometimes called the *antideformity position* [10]. The antideformity position has some variations that depend on the specific patient as well as the philosophy of the attending physicians. The position includes placing the wrist anywhere from 20-degree extension to neutral, the metacarpophalangeal joints in maximum flexion, and the interphalangeal joints in full extension or slight flexion, with the thumb in close to maximum abduction and extension. The reason for this position is that the dorsum of the hand is usually burned more severely than the volar surface, or at least is subject to more deformity, because the skin on this surface is thinner and less protected by fatty subcutaneous tissue than the palm. Therefore, the position concentrates on keeping the dorsal skin stretched as much as possible.

The usual position of deformity (Fig. 1–21) will have the wrist in flexion or neutral (as seen in the illustration), and the metacarpophalangeal joints in extension (sometimes hyperextension) [10]. The proximal interphalangeal joints flex, pulling the distal interphalangeal joints into extension or hyperextension due to the volar slippage of the lateral extensor tendons and the stretching of the dorsal retinacular ligaments [11]. The thumb is also pulled into a deformed position of adduction and external rotation [10].

References

1. American Academy of Orthopaedic Surgeons. *Atlas of Orthotics*. St. Louis: Mosby, 1975.
2. Anderson, M. H. *Upper Extremity Orthotics*. Springfield, Ill.: Thomas, 1965.
3. Blauvelt, C. T., and Nelson, F. Classifications of Fractures and Dislocations. Musculoskeletal Diseases and Related Terms. In *A Manual of Orthopaedic Terminology*. St. Louis: Mosby, 1977.
4. Gardner, E., Gray, D. J., O'Rahilly, R. *Anatomy* (2nd ed.). Philadelphia: Saunders, 1966. Pp. 181–201.
5. Hollis, L. I. Hand Rehabilitation. In H. L. Hopkins and H. D. Smith (Eds.), *Willard and Spackman's Occupational Therapy* (5th ed.). Philadelphia: Lippincott, 1978. P. 564.
6. Johnson, M. K. *The Hand Book*. Springfield, Ill.: Thomas, 1973.
7. Johnson, M. K., and Cohen, M. J. *The Hand Atlas*. Springfield, Ill.: Thomas, 1975.
8. Malick, M. H. *Manual on Dynamic Hand Splinting with Thermoplastic Materials*. Pittsburgh: Harmarville Rehabilitation Center, 1974. Pp. 19–41.
9. Quiring, D. P., and Warfel, J. H. *The Extremities* (3rd ed.). Philadelphia: Lea and Febiger, 1967.
10. Von Prince, K. M. P., and Yeakel, M. H. *The Splinting of Burn Patients*. Springfield, Ill.: Thomas, 1974. Pp. 32, 41–45.
11. Wynn Parry, C. B. *Rehabilitation of the Hand* (3rd ed.). London: Butterworth, 1973.

Suggested Reading

American Academy of Orthopaedic Surgeons. *Atlas of Orthotics*. St. Louis: Mosby, 1975.

Anderson, M. H. *Upper Extremity Orthotics*. Springfield, Ill.: Thomas, 1965.

Barr, N. *The Hand: Principles and Techniques of Simple Splintmaking in Rehabilitation*. Boston: Butterworth, 1975.

Blauvelt, C. T., and Nelson, F. *A Manual of Orthopaedic Terminology*. St. Louis: Mosby, 1977. Chapters 1 and 2.

Boyes, J. H. *Bunnell's Surgery of the Hand* (5th ed.). Philadelphia: Lippincott, 1970.

Byrne, J. J. *The Hand: Its Anatomy and Diseases*. Springfield, Ill.: Thomas, 1959.

Cailliet, R. *Hand Pain and Impairment* (2nd ed.). Philadelphia: Davis, 1976.

Capener, N. The hand in surgery. *J. Bone Joint Surg.* 38(1):128, 1956.

Carl, T. K. B. Unpublished data, 1971. Revised by M. E. Fess, and J. H. Kiel, 1973.

Gardner, E., Gray, D. J., O'Rahilly, R. *Anatomy* (2nd ed.). Philadelphia: Saunders, 1966. Pp. 181–201.

Hollis, L. I. Hand Rehabilitation. In H. L. Hopkins and H. D. Smith (Eds.), *Willard and Spackman's Occupational Therapy* (5th ed.). Philadelphia: Lippincott, 1978.

Institute and Workshop on Hand Splinting Construction. Pittsburgh: Harmarville Rehabilitation Center, March 9–11, June 2, 1967.

Johnson, M. K. *The Hand Book.* Springfield, Ill.: Thomas, 1973.

Johnson, M. K., and Cohen, M. J. *The Hand Atlas.* Springfield, Ill.: Thomas, 1975.

Malick, M. H. *Manual on Static Hand Splinting* (2nd ed.). Pittsburgh: Harmarville Rehabilitation Center, 1972.

Malick, M. H. *Manual on Dynamic Hand Splinting with Thermoplastic Materials.* Pittsburgh: Harmarville Rehabilitation Center, 1974.

Malick, M. H. Upper Extremity Orthotics. In H. L. Hopkins and H. D. Smith (Eds.), *Willard and Spackman's Occupational Therapy* (5th ed.). Philadelphia: Lippincott, 1978.

Moore, J. C. *Adaptive Equipment and Appliances.* Ann Arbor, Mich.: Overbeck, 1962.

O'Connor, J. R. Medical Aspects of Splinting. In E. R. Mayerson (Ed.), *Splinting Theory and Fabrication.* Clarence Center, New York: Goodrich Printing and Lithographers, 1971.

Quiring, D. P., and Warfel, J. H. *The Extremities* (3rd ed.). Philadelphia: Lea and Febiger, 1967.

Rasch, P. J., and Burke, R. K. *Kinesiology and Applied Anatomy* (6th ed.). Philadelphia: Lea and Febiger, 1978.

Thompson, C. W. *Kranz Manual of Kinesiology* (5th ed.). St. Louis: Mosby, 1965.

Von Prince, K. M. P., and Yeakel, M. H. *The Splinting of Burn Patients.* Springfield, Ill.: Thomas, 1974. Pp. 32, 41–45.

Wynn Parry, C. B. *Rehabilitation of the Hand* (3rd ed.). London: Butterworth, 1973.

The main purpose of splinting is to help the patient perform skills that are essential to daily life. When using a splint, one of the following justifications should apply: (1) support or immobilization of a body part, (2) correction or prevention of deformity, or (3) assistance or restoration of function [5].

If a splint is to accomplish its purpose, its design must take into consideration the functional ability of the entire extremity. A splint designed for wrist stabilization and finger flexion cannot be useful if the shoulder girdle masculature is insufficient to allow for hand placement.

Levers and Forces

When a joint is functioning normally, there are forces that affect its movement (or lack of movement) and permit a person to complete activities in a coordinated, controlled fashion. Some of these forces are the muscles and tendons that create movement, ligaments and connective tissues that keep all the parts in their correct positions, and weight of the body part as affected by gravity. All of these forces are perfectly balanced in the normal hand, permitting strong or delicate movements with little conscious effort.

In the event of an injury or illness, these forces can lose the balance that permits normal function. This balance can also be upset by such forces as spasticity or contractures.

When there is an imbalance of internal forces, a splint is an external force that can be used to compensate for this imbalance and improve or restore normal function. In order to accomplish this, the force of the splint must exceed the abnormal internal force. This force can cause problems, however, in the form of pressure sores in the delicate tissues that compose the arm. The ultimate goal must be to use a splint to maintain and improve the patient's comfort while increasing function [1].

In its broadest sense, a splint is a lever with three points of pressure that create a force acting on the arm. Figure 2–1 shows how three points of pressure are used in a lever to manipulate a large object. These three points of pressure in a splint are potential problem areas because they must push on the patient's skin in order to apply a force to the problem area. Figure 2–2 shows the points of pressure placed in a simple cock-up splint.

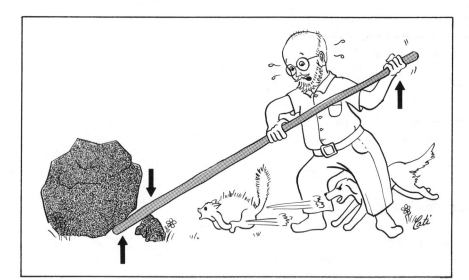

Figure 2-1. Use of a lever to move a heavy rock.

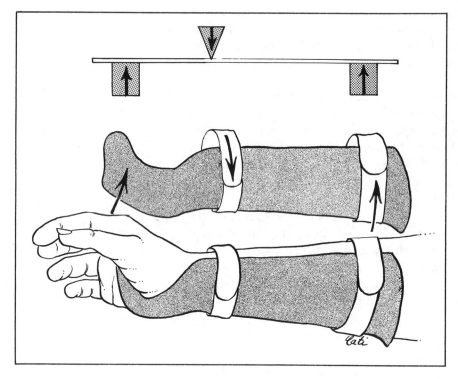

Figure 2-2. Location of the three points of pressure in a simple cock-up splint.

Anyone applying splints to a patient must recognize the biomechanical principles of levers, while providing a splint that allows for function without creating discomfort or damage from too much pressure on the patient's skin. The rules that must be considered are

1. Design the lever arms of the splint as long as possible in order to displace the pressure necessary to create the required force.
2. If an unsplinted joint is to be allowed motion, the splint must not extend into the defined boundaries of that joint (including the skin creases).
3. The axis point of pressure of the splint (lever) must always be exactly over the axis of the joint being splinted.
4. Be sure all three points of pressure are present and in the proper location.
5. The points of pressure of the splint must be made as wide as possible on the patient's arm to disperse the pressure over the skin and decrease the chance of a pressure sore.

6. The splint should allow for normal anatomical properties. These include placement in a functional position, support of the arches of the hand, allowance for dual obliquity, and allowance for all possible prehension patterns, given the design of the specific splint being used.

Splint Design

After determining the extent of the patient's problem and where an external force is needed to correct the problem, a decision about the design of the splint must be made. Usually splints are designed to be either dorsal or volar. This means that the major portion of the splint is positioned on either the dorsal or the volar surface of the hand and/or forearm with very little of the splint on the opposite surface. Figure 2–3 shows a dorsal splint (right) that stabilizes the wrist and maintains the web space, along with a volar splint (left) that has the same purpose.

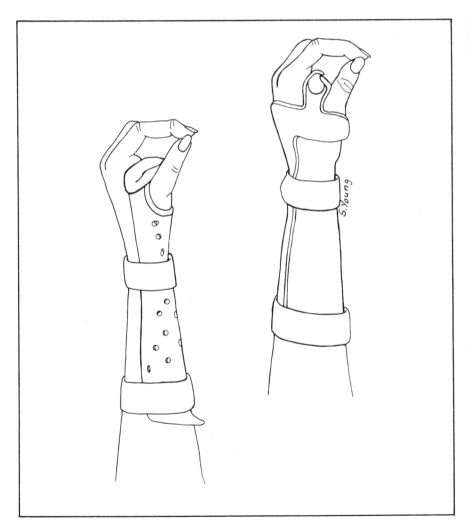

Figure 2-3. A dorsal splint and a volar splint, both accomplishing the same purpose.

The decision to make a dorsal or a volar splint depends on the patient problem, the particular parts needed in the splint to correct that problem, and the preferences of the physician, therapist, and patient involved. Volar splinting has the advantage of firm comfortable support with pressure distributed well [4]. The two major disadvantages are that the palm is obstructed and that it is more difficult to add attachment parts. The dorsal type splint allows the palm to be left more open to sensation, and any necessary attachments are usually easier to add. For these reasons, the dorsal splint is often the base for dynamic splints. The therapist making the splint will find, however, that it is more difficult to distribute pressure evenly with a splint that has a dorsal design.

Another design decision is whether the splint should be static or dynamic. A static splint has no movable parts and allows no motion in the joint or joints being splinted. Hazards that can result from static splinting for too long, or without an accompanying exercise program, are disuse atrophy, stiffness, and dependency [2]. It has been reported that static splinting may be contraindicated in cases of hypertonicity [3].

Cailliet [2] has described what he calls semidynamic splints. These splints have no movable parts, but provide function by positioning one or more joints in a more favorable position. An example of this is a simple cock-up splint, which positions the wrist in extension and permits the fingers to function more effectively. A splint placing the thumb in abduction and opposition, thereby permitting prehension, is also an example of semidynamic splinting.

Dynamic splinting (also called functional, kinetic, active, or lively) is the use of movable parts, usually attached to a static splint base. The dynamic splint applies a force to a body part and permits movement of certain joints. Functionally it guides the movement, prevents unwanted movement, and can even actively move or resist certain movements [2]. The source of power for a dynamic splint may be either internal (the patient's muscles) or external (rubber bands, wires, cords, springs, elastic, and sometimes an electronic or a pneumatic unit).

Parts of Splints

While making decisions about the design of a splint, one must also remember that a splint can be put together in many different ways. There are, however, some universally recognized parts that are used in splints. Some of these parts can be added in a variety of ways, while others will at least partially determine whether the splint will be dorsal or volar, static or dynamic. The following list describes most of these parts and illustrates the different ways in which they can be used. An attempt has been made to show the possible variations in the parts.

1. The *transverse metacarpal arch support (palmar arch support)* is the portion of a splint covering the volar surface of the metacarpal area of the hand. The part must be curved to provide support for the anatomical arch (Fig. 2–4).

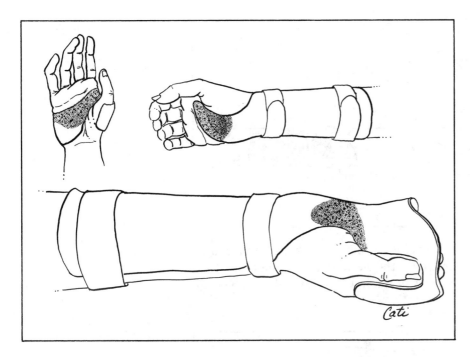

Figure 2-4. Transverse metacarpal arch support.

2. A *wrist extensor bar* is any portion of the splint covering the wrist area (dorsal or volar), stabilizing the wrist in any position; desired position is usually extension (Fig. 2–5).

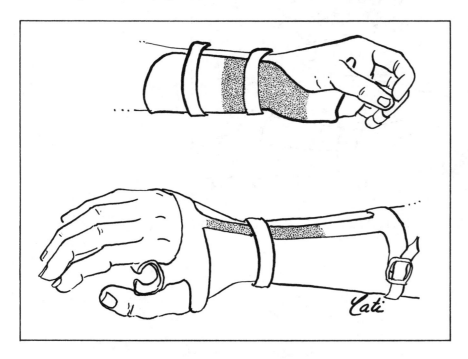

Figure 2-5. Wrist extensor bar.

3. The *forearm bar* is the portion of a splint covering the forearm, dorsal or volar. It provides a long lever arm to help disperse the amount of pressure exerted on the hand and arm. Usually this piece is two-thirds the length of the forearm to maintain motion of the elbow (Fig. 2–6).

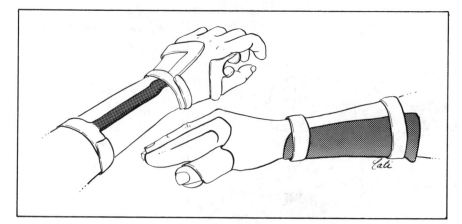

Figure 2-6. Forearm bar.

4. The **C** *bar* is a curved piece that holds the metacarpal bones of the thumb and index finger apart to maintain the web space between them. Flexion of the interphalangeal joints of the index finger and thumb are allowed (Fig. 2–7).

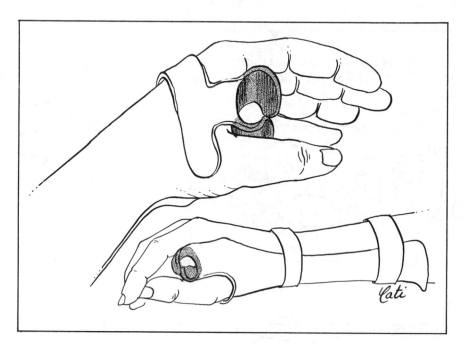

Figure 2-7. **C** *bar.*

5. The *thumb post* stabilizes the joints of the thumb in a position that allows opposition with the other four fingers (Fig. 2–8).

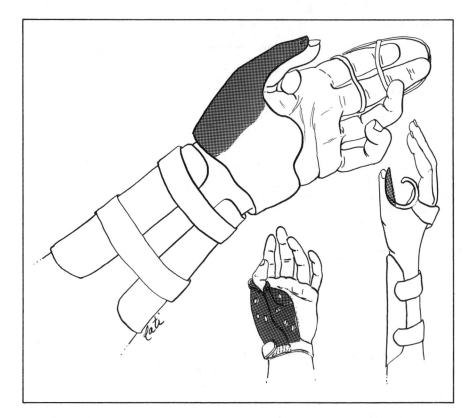

Figure 2-8. Thumb post.

6. An *opponens bar* is a small piece on the dorsal surface of the first metacarpal that stabilizes it, volar to the second metacarpal bone so that opposition and prehension are possible (Fig. 2–9).

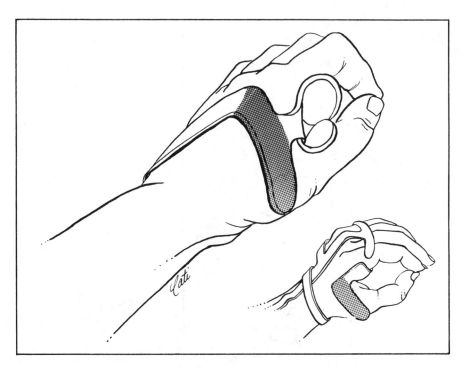

Figure 2-9. Opponens bar.

7. The *finger pan (platform)* supports all the joints of the second through fifth fingers, usually in slight flexion, as seen in the longitudinal arch of the functional position. It eliminates all finger movement to provide rest for the fingers or to prevent or correct finger contractures (Fig. 2–10).

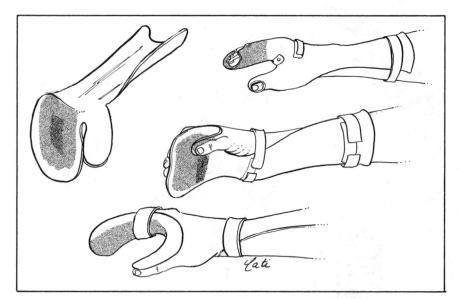

Figure 2-10. Finger pan.

8. A *hypothenar bar* is used in a dorsal splint only. It is the part that extends around the ulnar side of the hand to the volar surface and holds the splint in place on the ulnar side. It supports the fourth and fifth metacarpal area of the transverse arch, and it may prevent ulnar deviation of the wrist if attached to a splint that has a forearm bar (Fig. 2–11).

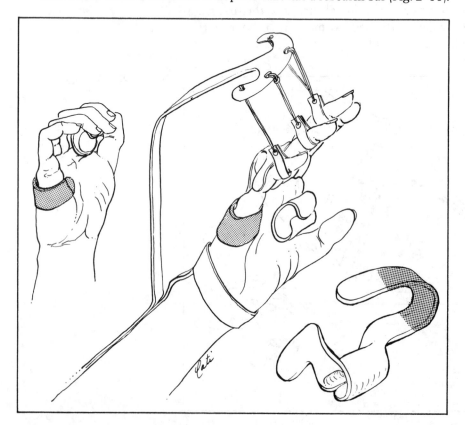

Figure 2-11. Hypothenar bar.

9. The *lumbrical bar* rests on the dorsal surface of the proximal phalanges, serving to prevent hyperextension of the MP joints. This part is seldom seen on a volar splint (Fig. 2–12).

Figure 2-12. Lumbrical bar.

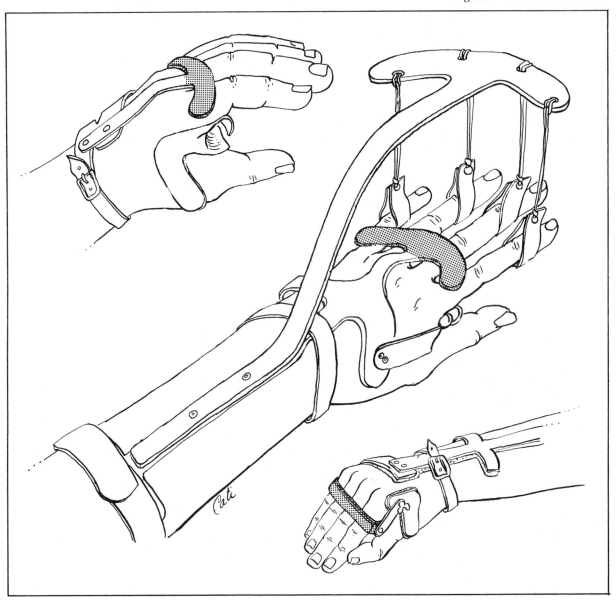

10. The *dorsal metacarpal bar* extends across the dorsal surface of the meta-carpal bones. It must have a curve that approximates the transverse arch on the dorsal surface. It provides a centrally located place to attach distal, proximal, radial, and ulnar parts of a dorsal splint (Fig. 2–13).

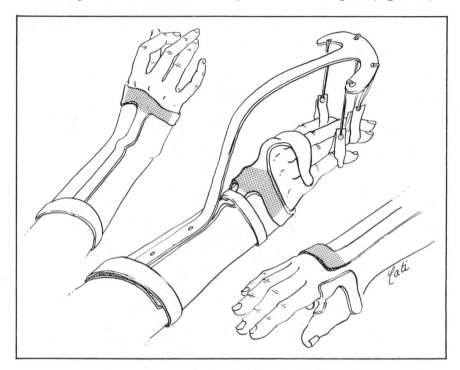

Figure 2-13. Dorsal meta-carpal bar.

11. The *deviation bar* is an extension on the sides of a splint, usually in the metacarpal or phalangeal area, to prevent radial or ulnar deviation in any joint covered by the splint part (Fig. 2–14).

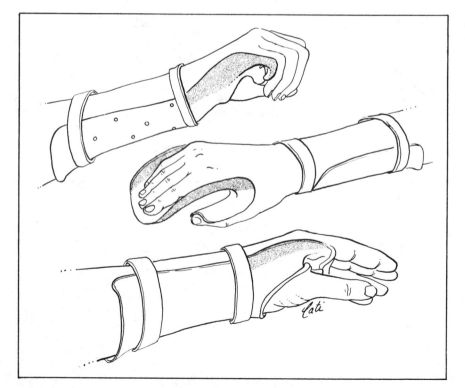

Figure 2-14. Deviation bar.

12. A *reinforcement or stabilization bar* is anything (including extra width or length, extension from a part, or a whole new part) whose only purpose is to maintain the splint in the proper position, either by strengthening it or stabilizing it (Fig. 2–15). This includes a *cross bar*, which is placed at the proximal end of a dorsal forearm bar to keep the splint from deviating on the forearm (Fig. 2–16).

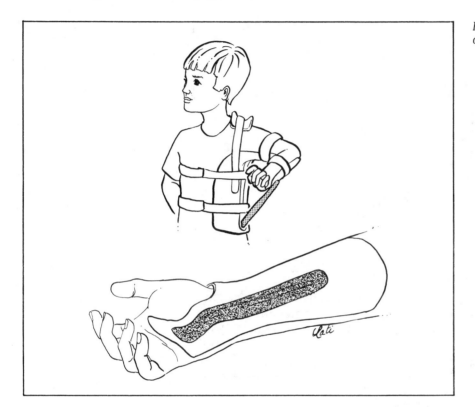

Figure 2-15. Reinforcement or stabilization bar.

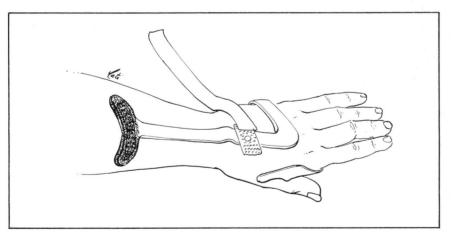

Figure 2-16. Cross bar.

13. A *miscellaneous equipment attachment* (Fig. 2–17) is anything added to a splint that provides a specific function (e.g., an attachment to hold a pencil or comb or as shown, a universal cuff to hold a fork or spoon).

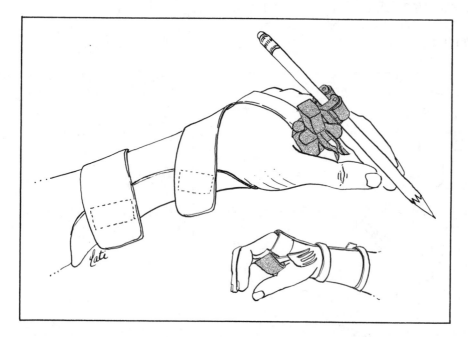

Figure 2-17. Miscellaneous equipment attachment.

14. A *prop* is an attachment on the volar surface of a hand splint designed to hold the arm off any surface in order to prevent pressure. This can easily be adapted to prevent pressure on body parts other than the hand (Fig. 2–18).

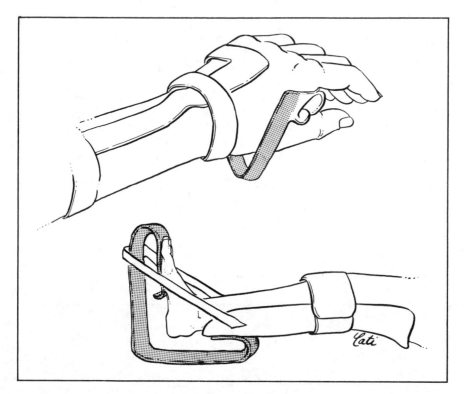

Figure 2-18. Prop.

15. *Connector bars* are small sections of splinting material positioned between functional parts to space these parts in their proper relationship pencil or comb or, as shown, a universal cuff to hold a fork or spoon).

Figure 2-19. Connector bars.

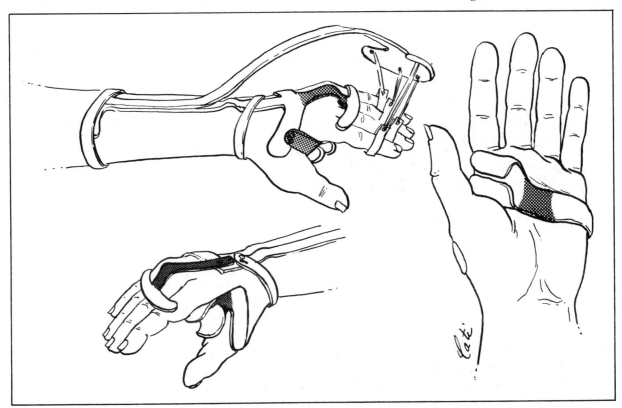

16. *Straps and closures* are used to hold the splint in place on the arm and to fasten it securely (Fig. 2–20).

Figure 2-20. Straps and closures.

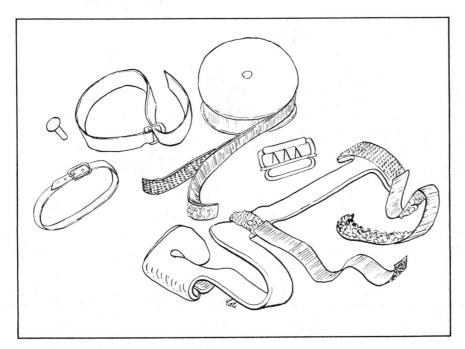

17. *Dynamic assist* (Fig. 2-21) is any part or material added to a splint that makes it movable (e.g., elastic, rubber bands, dental dam, spring wire, or a mobile joint).

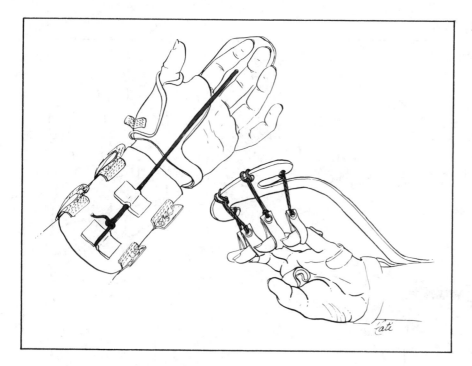

Figure 2-21. Dynamic assist.

18. An *outrigger (dynamic extension assist* or *dynamic finger extension assist)* extends from a splint, holding dynamic assists, which help in flexion or extension of the fingers (Fig. 2–22). Another type is a *dorsal interosseous bar*, a piece extending from the splint beside the index or small finger to provide or assist abduction of the finger (Fig. 2–23).

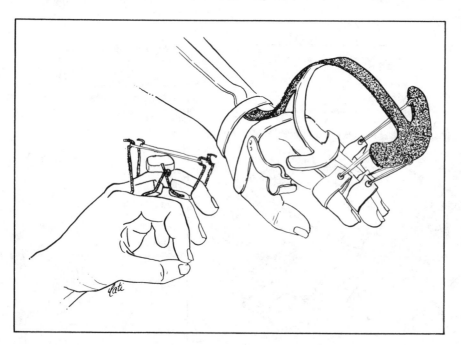

Figure 2-22. Outrigger.

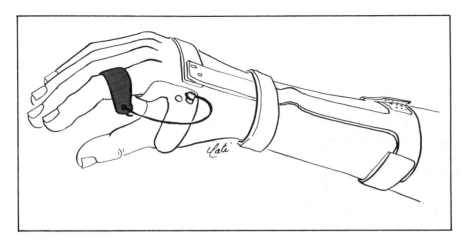

Figure 2-23. Dorsal interosseous bar.

19. *Finger and thumb loops* are small rings of leather, plastic, metal, or fabric made to fit a finger and attached to rubber bands or other dynamic assists so that the finger can be assisted in the desired function. Its purpose is to widen that point of pressure to prevent the formation of decubiti (Fig. 2–24).

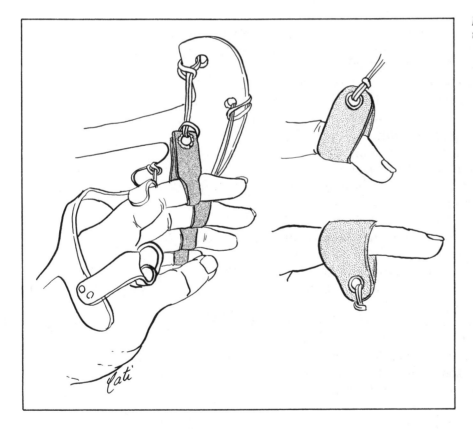

Figure 2-24. Finger and thumb loops.

In order to understand how a therapist uses the knowledge of splint parts, read the following example.

Mr. X has sustained an injury to his right hand, which has caused weakened wrist extensors and tightness of his thumb web space. The doctor wants the wrist positioned in 15-degree extension in order to prevent further stretching of the extensor musculature. This wrist position will also allow better finger function. In addition, the doctor wants the web space protected from further contracture while being stretched back to normal.

The two parts needed in the splint are a **C** bar and a wrist extensor bar. In order for these to work, however, other parts must be added, and the selection of these parts depends on the choice made by the patient, therapist, and doctor. The splint shown in Figure 3–16 would fill the requirement. If the simple cock-up splint with **C** bar attachment (see Fig. 3–16) is chosen, the additional parts needed are

1. A forearm bar to help disperse the pressure caused by placing the wrist in extension
2. A transverse metacarpal arch support, since the splint must cross the palm of the hand and therefore support the arch
3. Straps and closures that will hold the splint in place

If the splint in Figure 3–16 is not strong enough, or if a type of plastic not suitable for that splint is used, then the splint shown in Figure 3–27 might be preferable. The cock-up splint with a rolled **C** bar (see Fig. 3–27) requires all the previously mentioned parts, plus radial and ulnar deviation bars. In this case, the deviation bars add contour to the stretchy plastic that must be used, make the splint stronger, and add even more stability to the patient's hand, which may or may not be desirable.

Another option is a dorsal splint, and again there are two choices. The splint shown in Figure 3–37 is one option. The Warm Springs long opponens splint (see Fig. 3–37) has a **C** bar, a wrist extensor bar, and a dorsal forearm bar. In addition, this splint requires

1. An opponens bar, which stabilizes the thumb metacarpal in opposition and also stabilizes the radial side of the hand in the splint
2. A hypothenar bar, which stabilizes the ulnar side of the hand in the splint while it supports the fourth and fifth metacarpals in the correct position for the transverse metacarpal arch
3. A dorsal metacarpal bar that connects all the parts on the dorsal surface and is curved in the shape of the transverse metacarpal arch
4. A connector bar between the **C** bar and opponens bar to hold them in the correct relationship to each other
5. A cross bar to stabilize the dorsal forearm bar

If this splint is selected, the transverse metacarpal arch is supported indirectly by the **C** bar and the hypothenar bar with a small space between these two parts.

If a dorsal splint is desired, but direct support of the transverse metacarpal arch is preferable, then the splint shown in Figure 3–38 is necessary. The Rancho long opponens splint has all the parts mentioned for the first dorsal splint, plus a connector bar between the **C** bar and the hypothenar bar that will provide direct support to the arch. In order to allow the splint enough flexibility to be removed, a space must be put between the dorsal metacarpal bar and the **C** bar, opponens bar combination.

A therapist need not list all the parts of the splint for various options, nor necessarily offer all of the options to the doctor or patient. Part of the decision should be based on the type of splint the therapist makes best and whether the plastic is available for the specific splint.

It is helpful, however, for the novice to realize that to solve one problem there are several options to choose from, each incorporating the same basic splint parts, although the appearance of the splint is quite different.

References

1. Anderson, M. H. *Upper Extremity Orthotics.* Springfield, Ill.: Thomas, 1965.
2. Cailliet, R. *Hand Pain and Impairment* (2nd ed.). Philadelphia: Davis, 1976.
3. Farber, S. D. *Neurorehabilitation: A Multisensory Approach.* Philadelphia: Saunders, 1982.
4. O'Connor, J. R. Medical Aspects of Splinting. In E. R. Mayerson (Ed.), *Splinting Theory and Fabrication.* Clarence Center, N.Y.: Goodrich, 1971.
5. Smith, E. M., and Juvinall, R. C. Mechanics of Bracing. In S. Licht (Ed.), *Orthotics Etcetera.* Baltimore: Waverly, 1966.

Suggested Reading

American Occupational Therapy Association. Occupational therapy: Its definition and function. *Am. J. Occup. Ther.* 26:204, 1972.

Anderson, M. H. *Upper Extremity Orthotics.* Springfield, Ill.: Thomas, 1965.

Blauvelt, C. T., and Nelson, F. *A Manual of Orthopaedic Terminology.* St. Louis: Mosby, 1977.

Burkman, E., et al. *The Natural World.* Morristown, N.J.: Silver Burdett, 1975.

Byrne, J. J. *The Hand: Its Anatomy and Diseases.* Springfield, Ill.: Thomas, 1959.

Cailliet, R. *Hand Pain and Impairment* (2nd ed.). Philadelphia: Davis, 1976.

Carl, T. K. B. Unpublished data, 1971. Revised by M. E. Fess and J. H. Kiel, 1973.

Crutchfield, C. A., and Barnes, M. R. *Neurophysiological Basis of Patient Treatment: The Muscle Spindle, Vol. 1.* Morgantown, W.V.: Stokesville, 1973.

Farber, S. D. *Neurorehabilitation: A Multisensory Approach.* Philadelphia: Saunders, 1982.

Institute and Workshop on Hand Splinting Construction. Pittsburgh: Harmarville Rehabilitation Center, March 9–11, June 2, 1967.

Malick, M. H. *Manual on Static Hand Splinting* (2nd ed.). Pittsburgh: Harmarville Rehabilitation Center, 1972.

Malick, M. H. *Manual on Dynamic Hand Splinting with Thermoplastic Materials.* Pittsburgh: Harmarville Rehabilitation Center, 1974.

Moore, J. C. *Adaptive Equipment and Appliances.* Ann Arbor, Mich.: Overbeck, 1962.

Nickel, V. L., Perry, J., and Snelson, B. *Handbook of Handsplints.* Downey, Calif.: Rancho Los Amigos Hospital.

O'Connor, J. R. Medical Aspects of Splinting. In E. R. Mayerson (Ed.), *Splinting Theory and Fabrication.* Clarence Center, N.Y.: Goodrich, 1971.

Orthotic Systems. P.O. Box 20262, Houston, Texas 77025, February, 1969.

Smith, E. M., and Juvinall, R. C. *Mechanics of Bracing.* In S. Licht (Ed.), *Orthotics Etcetera.* Baltimore: Waverley, 1966.

3. Designing a Pattern for a Splint

There are several ways to obtain a pattern for a splint, including tracing the pattern from a book. Although this is easy, the patterns seldom fit a patient properly. The problem seems to be that hands, especially injured hands, do not come in a standard shape or in standard sizes. A solution to the problem, and a second way to obtain a pattern, is to adapt the patterns found in books. This, if done correctly, can be quite successful, provided the book is available when needed. Another way to get a pattern is to make an original for each patient. There are several techniques for doing this, some quite effective and some often resulting in a poor fit caused by inconsistent use of concrete and anatomical data.

Following are directions for making original patterns for four common, static splints.

1. Simple cock-up splint
2. Cock-up splint with a rolled **C** bar
3. Resting pan splint
4. Long and short opponens splints

The directions are based on anatomical landmarks and very specific measurements, including references to special considerations in forming a splint from the pattern.

The necessary materials for making most splinting patterns are paper towels, pencil, scissors, masking tape, ruler, a skin or grease (china marking) pencil (optional), and occasionally a positive mold. (See p. 101 for further description and directions.)

Volar Splints

Directions for making a forearm bar pattern for volar type splints:

1. Place pronated arm flat on a paper towel that has been opened and smoothed to one layer. The fingers should be flat and be approximately one-fourth inch apart at the distal end. The entire arm, from finger tips to elbow, should be resting on the paper towel (Fig. 3–1). The paper towel can be placed diagonally under the arm or taped to a second paper towel if it is not large enough for the arm being splinted.

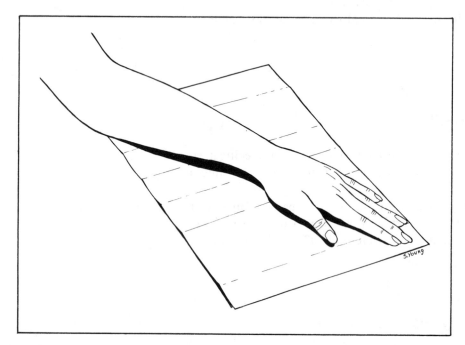

Figure 3-1. Place the pronated hand flat on a paper towel.

2. After being certain that the wrist and fingers are being held straight (i.e., not in ulnar or radial deviation), trace around the hand and arm to the elbow. Be sure when tracing around the arm that the pencil is held perpendicular to the table, so that the size of the arm will not be altered (Fig. 3–2A, B). It is not necessary to trace around each finger for these splints. Do not trace the thumb. Stop at the bottom of the web space, proximal to the head of the metacarpal (MC) of the index finger, then begin again at the base of the first MC. There will be an open space in the finished drawing where the thumb would have been (Fig. 3–3).

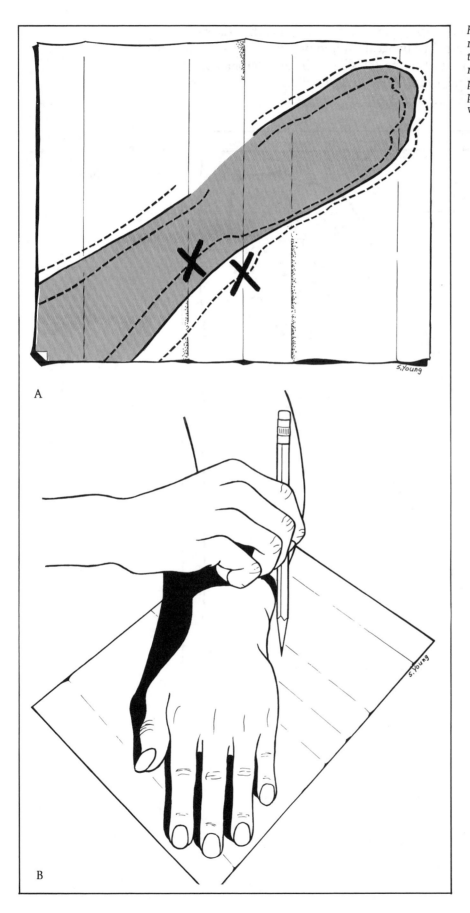

Figure 3-2. A. If the pencil is not held correctly while tracing the hand, the result may be the wrong size. B. The pencil must be held perpendicular to the paper towel while tracing the hand.

3. Without moving the hand, mark the axis of the wrist joint, the axis of the second and fifth metacarpal phalangeal (MP) joints, and both sides of the proximal interphalangeal joints (PIPs) and distal interphalangeal joints (DIPs) of the second, third, fourth, and fifth digits, and the desired proximal length of the splint (Fig. 3–3).

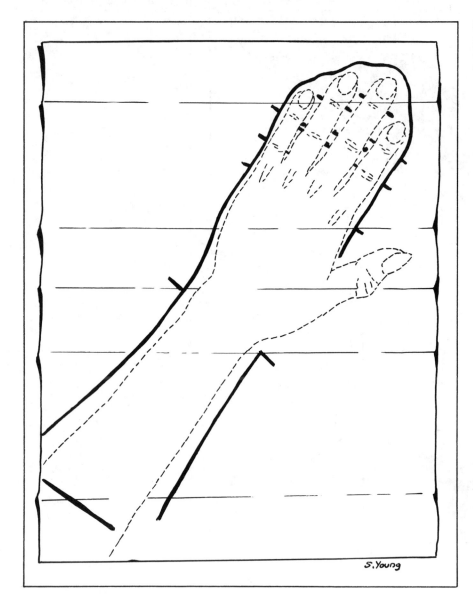

Figure 3-3. Mark the desired proximal length and the axis of all the joints. Do not trace around the thumb.

a. How to determine the desired proximal length of the splint: In order to provide the longest lever arm possible and still not obstruct elbow motion, splints usually extend onto the forearm two-thirds of the distance from the axis of the wrist joint to the elbow. This distance can be established by measuring with a ruler from the elbow to the axis of the wrist joint, then mathematically determining two-thirds of the distance. You will notice that if the olecranon process is used to determine the elbow rather than the flexion crease, the distance is longer. There will be a better result if the elbow flexion crease is used as the measuring point (Fig. 3–4). With some practice it is possible to estimate the length rather than using a ruler and determining it mathematically. The length of a completed forearm bar pattern should be checked by holding the pattern in place while the elbow is flexed to see that sufficient range of motion will be available with the splint in place.

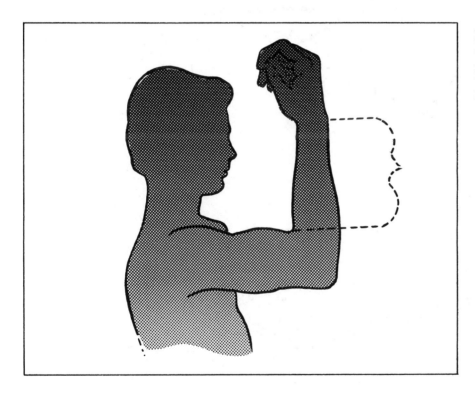

Figure 3-4. Measure the distance between the axis of the wrist joint and the elbow flexion crease when determining the length of the forearm bar.

4. Continuing to leave the arm stationary, tape the paper towel around the arm. It is helpful to tape the paper to the arm as well as to the paper itself (Fig. 3–5A, B).

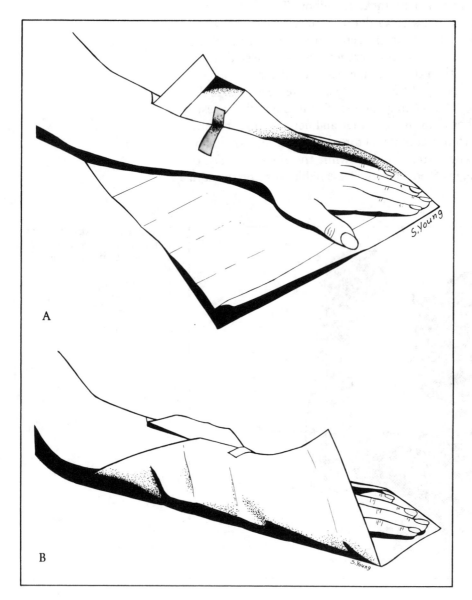

A

B

Figure 3-5A, B. Tape the paper towel around the arm.

5. Carefully hold onto the hand and paper towel, keeping the palm from sliding or rotating on the towel as you pick it up to look at the palmar surface. Trace the flexion crease and the thenar crease onto the paper towel.

a. Flexion crease: Keeping the thumb in an adducted, slightly extended position, have (or help) the patient flex the MP joints into 90-degree flexion. Attempt to keep the paper towel from wadding or folding in the palm. Draw a line on the flexion crease with the hand in this position.

Note: The flexion crease is neither the distal palmar crease nor the proximal palmar crease seen in Figure 1–6 (page 9), but a line that must not cross either the bony joint or the crease caused by that joint. The flexion crease will be some combination of these two lines (Fig. 3–6).

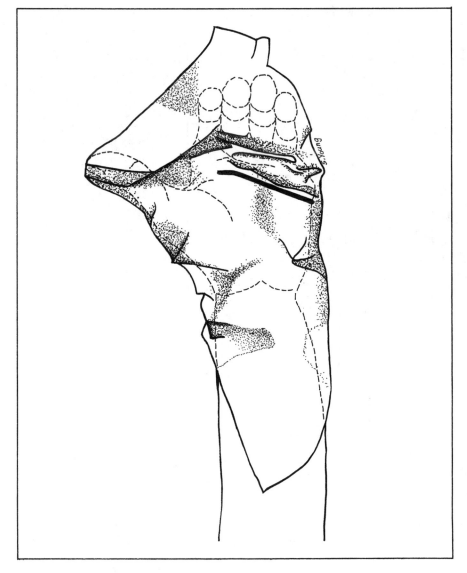

Figure 3-6. Mark the flexion crease.

b. Thenar crease: Have the patient hold all MP joints in full (180-degree) extension. Place the thumb in abduction. Trace the thenar crease. **Note:** The thenar crease is shown in Figure 1–6 (page 9). The line that is needed for making splints should stop at the point where it intersects the flexion crease (see 5.a); it should not extend through the web space (Fig. 3–7).

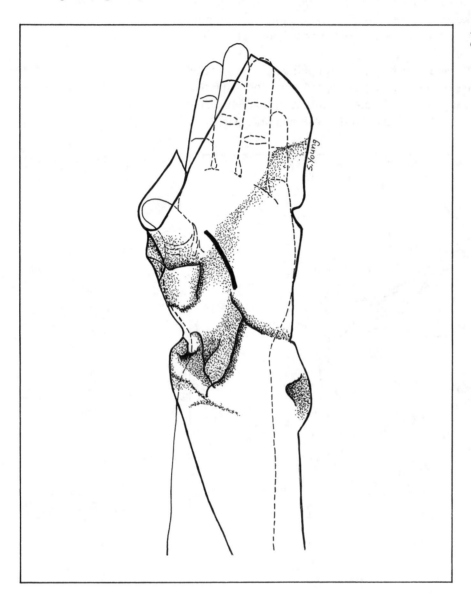

Figure 3-7. Mark the thenar crease.

6. Remove the paper towel from the patient's arm and transfer the markings that are currently on both sides of the paper towel to one side. It is usually easier to transfer the flexion cease and thenar crease lines rather than the entire tracing of the arm with all of the other notations (Fig. 3–8).
Note: At this point be sure that both the radial and ulnar ends of the flexion crease are proximal to the markings for the axis of the MP joints. If this is not the case, either go back and attempt to locate the problem or begin again.

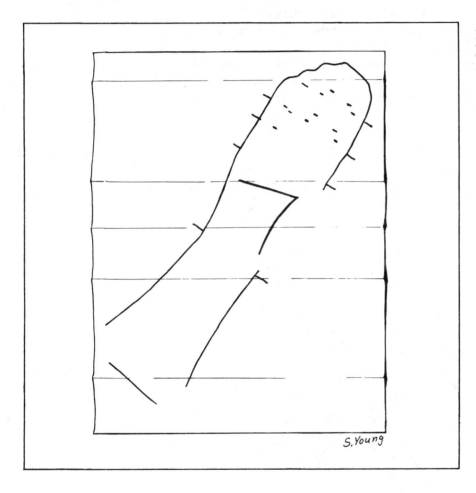

Figure 3-8. Transfer the flexion crease and thenar crease marks to the other side of the paper towel.

7. To provide sufficient curving contour in the forearm bar of the splint, add width to the sides of the forearm. Usually one-half of the distance up the sides of the forearm is a satisfactory width for a volar splint. To determine how much width to add, lay the forearm on a flat surface. Measure the thickness of the forearm from the flat surface to the top of the arm at a point one-half the distance between the elbow flexion crease and the axis of the wrist joint. Divide this measured distance by two and add the resulting measurement to each side of the traced forearm from the mark indicating the axis of the wrist joint to the mark indicating the correct length of the splint (Fig. 3–9). Again, with experience this distance can be estimated rather than figured mathematically.

Note: Frequently one corner of the pattern does not fit onto the paper towel. When this occurs, it can be corrected either when tracing the pattern onto the plastic, or by taping a small piece of paper towel where it is needed.

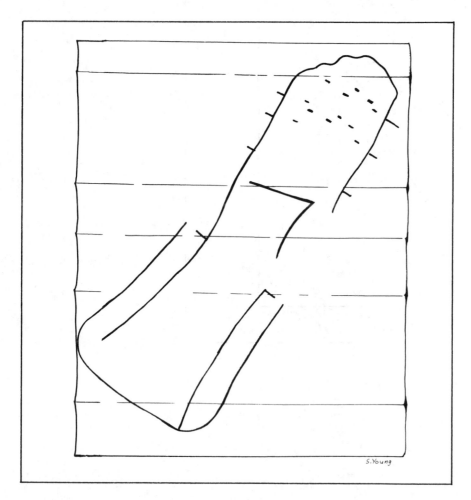

Figure 3-9. Draw the boundaries for the forearm bar.

8. Round the corners formed where the width lines and the length lines intersect. For aesthetic purposes be sure that the length lines look approximately even on each side of the forearm bar when measured from the axis of the wrist joint (Fig. 3–9).

The above eight steps will complete an accurate forearm bar pattern for most volar splints and will provide sufficient markings in the hand area to make any of the following three splints.

Simple Cock-up Splint
The purpose of a simple cock-up splint (Fig. 3–10) may be to prevent wrist flexion contractures, prevent overstretching weak extensor muscles, improve finger function, promote healing by immobilization, or provide support for a weakened joint structure.

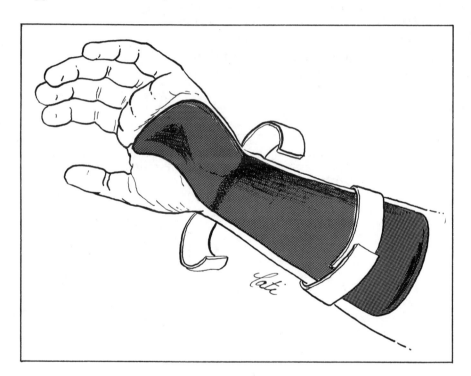

Figure 3-10. Simple cock-up splint.

Directions for making a simple cock-up splint pattern:

1. Complete the eight steps for making the forearm bar. See pages 44–53.
2. Round the point made at the intersection of the thenar crease and the flexion crease.
   Important: This intersection must be proximal to the MP joints and ulnar to the line tracing the radial side of the hand. Often the intersection of the two lines is in line with the dots that mark the PIP and DIP joints between the index and middle fingers.
3. Smoothly connect the proximal end of the thenar crease to the radial side of the forearm bar. This line must not leave any points on the radial side of the pattern that could cause pressure on the radial styloid process. In order to prevent this pressure, some width will have to be removed on the forearm bar proximal to the axis of the wrist joint (Fig. 3–11).
4. The ulnar end of the line drawn on the flexion crease should begin to curve proximally at the center of the fifth metacarpal bone on the volar surface but also continue ulnarly to the center of the ulnar border of the hand. Continue this line toward the wrist until it connects with the ulnar side of the forearm bar. Again, do not draw a point that could cause pressure on the side of the splint pattern (Fig. 3–11).

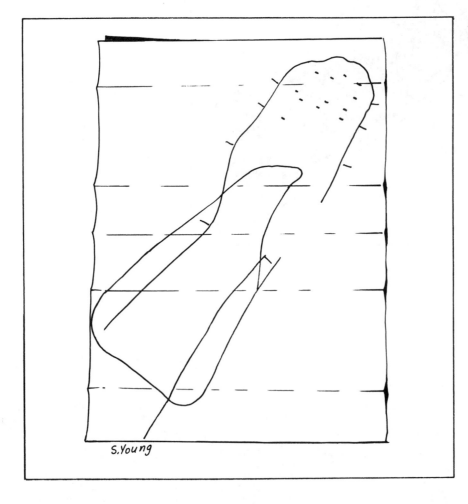

S.Young

Figure 3-11. Palmar portion of simple cock-up splint pattern attached to forearm bar.

5. Check the pattern for fit.

    a. Cut out the completed pattern and hold it in place on the patient's hand. Be sure that the wrist is in extension and that the pattern is in the intended position on the hand. The edges of the splint pattern at the flexion crease and at the thenar crease should be on their respective creases. The forearm bar should be straight on the patient's forearm.

    b. Check the following areas.

        (1) Flexion crease: The pattern must extend to the flexion crease on the hand; it may touch, but not cover, it. The MP joints must not be obstructed in flexion.

        (2) Thenar crease: The pattern must extend to the thenar crease on the hand, but not cover it. The thumb must not be obstructed as it abducts or attempts opposition.

        (3) Width of forearm bar: It should come halfway up either side of the forearm. It must not begin to wrap around onto the dorsal side of the arm or the splint will be difficult to put on and take off.

        (4) Length of forearm bar: It should extend proximally on the forearm two-thirds of the distance from the axis of the wrist joint to the elbow flexion crease. The elbow must be allowed to flex and extend without creating pressure either on the forearm or on the upper arm.

(5) Pressure should not be created over either of the styloid processes. The splint pattern can partially cover these areas, with the intention of bending the plastic out with a small lip away from these bony prominences where necessary. In an attempt to prevent this pressure, *do not* curve in the sides of the splint pattern, making the wrist area very narrow and weak (Fig. 3–12).

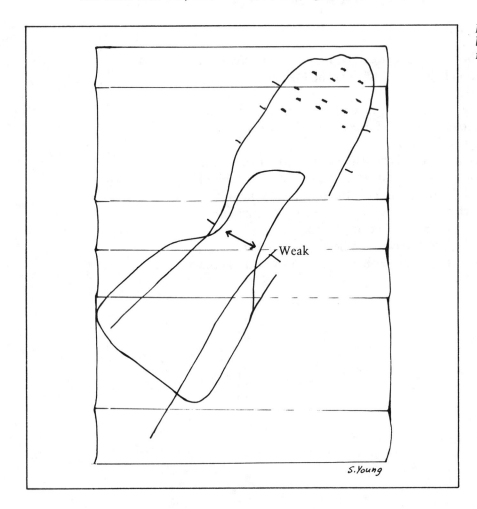

Weak

S. Young

Figure 3-12. The splint will be weak if the pattern is too narrow in the wrist area.

(6) Deviation: Be sure that the pattern is straight and will not hold the wrist in radial or ulnar deviation. If the pattern appears to deviate when it is flat, check it on the patient before altering it, as it may not support the wrist in incorrect alignment when it is on the arm.

Ulnar Deviation Bar. The ulnar deviation bar, **C** bar, connector bar, and opponens bar are static attachment parts that can be used with a simple cock-up splint. The purpose of this ulnar deviation bar (Fig. 3–13) is to prevent or correct ulnar deviation of the wrist.

The pattern for this attachment can be drawn into the original pattern by extending the ulnar side to fit the proper dimensions, or it can be added by taping a small piece of paper towel to the side of the splint pattern, then drawing the proper dimensions.

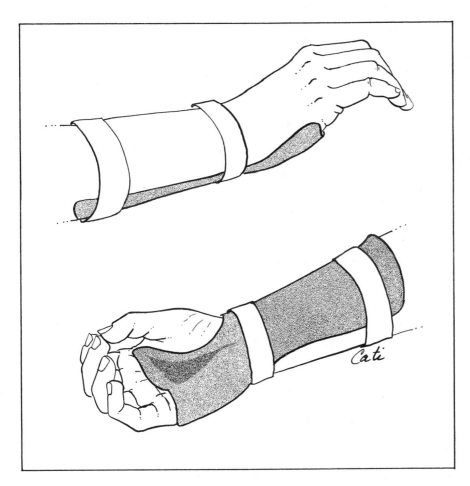

Figure 3-13. Simple cock-up splint with ulnar deviation bar attachment.

Note: When tracing the pattern for a simple cock-up splint with this attachment onto the plastic, the ulnar deviation bar is *always* part of the original splint. It would be a potential source of pressure sores if it were added to the splint as an attachment. Directions for making the ulnar deviation bar pattern:

1. Hold or tape a completed pattern for a simple cock-up splint in place on the hand. This pattern must be either not yet cut out, or it must have a small piece of paper (about two inches by four inches) taped onto the distal end of the ulnar side of the splint.
2. Beginning toward the middle or ulnar end of the flexion crease, extend this line around the ulnar side of the hand to the edge of the dorsal surface. This line must be as far distal as possible so that the length of the lever arm will minimize pressure, but it must be low enough to remain proximal to the fifth metacarpal head to allow for flexion of the MP joint. It also must not be so wide that it goes onto the dorsal surface.
3. Beginning at the ulnar end of the line draw a line along the length of the fifth metacarpal toward the wrist tapering it into the ulnar side of the original splint. There should be no additional width proximal to the axis of the wrist joint. Figure 3–14 shows the general shape of a pattern for a simple cock-up splint with an ulnar deviation bar attachment that has been laid flat.

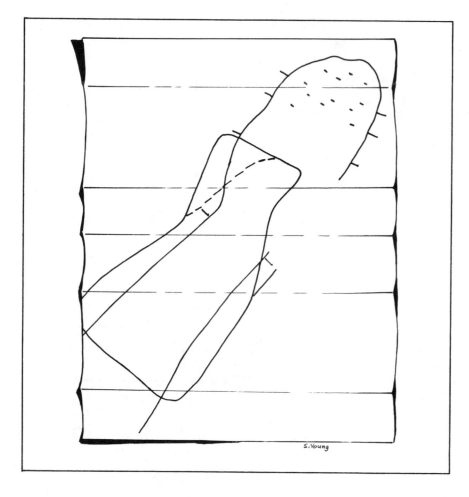

Figure 3-14. Pattern for a simple cock-up splint with an ulnar deviation bar attachment.

S. Young

4. Check the ulnar deviation bar pattern for fit.

   a. Be sure the flexion of the fifth MP joint is not hampered when the pattern is held in place on the hand. The pattern must reach the flexion crease, and must also be proximal to the head of the fifth metacarpal on the volar and ulnar sides.

   b. On the ulnar side the pattern should not extend onto the dorsal surface. This will assure prevention of ulnar deviation, but will not make the splint difficult to put on the hand.

   c. As the attachment part tapers into the original splint the line should be smooth and streamlined. It should look like part of the splint rather than like something has been added. This is important to prevent weakness and also for the aesthetic quality of the splint. Compare Figure 3–15 with the correct shape shown in Figure 3–14.

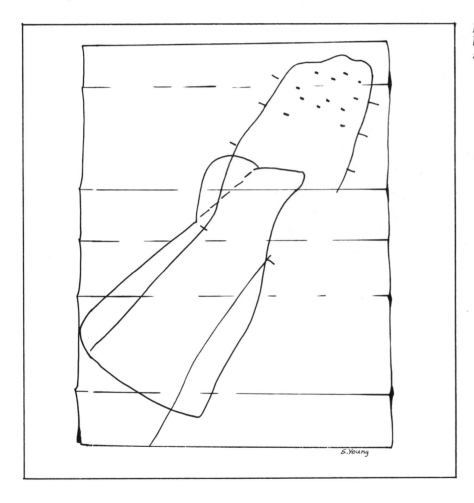

Figure 3-15. Ulnar deviation bar attached incorrectly to a simple cock-up splint.

C *Bar.* The purpose of a **C** bar is to maintain the web space between the thumb and index finger (Fig. 3–16).

The pattern for this attachment must be drawn separately from the original pattern.

Note: When the splint with this attachment is drawn on plastic to make the final splint, it is always *part* of the main pattern. It would be a potential source of pressure sores if it were added to the splint as an attachment. Directions for making the **C** bar pattern:

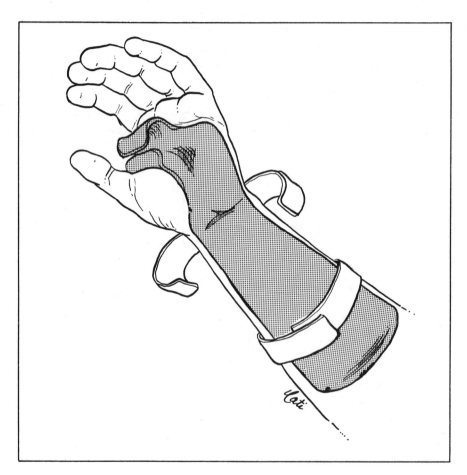

*Figure 3-16. Simple cock-up splint with **C** bar attachment.*

1. Length: Have or help the patient hold the hand to be splinted in a functional position. Using a strip of paper towel (about three inches by six inches) measure from the edge of the PIP joint of the index finger to the edge of the IP joint of the thumb. Do not allow the paper towel to cover these joints. While doing this the paper towel must be smooth against the web space (i.e., without wrinkles or gaps). Fold and crease the paper towel so that its measurements are within the stated boundaries. Cut off the excess paper towel that has been folded down (Fig. 3–17).

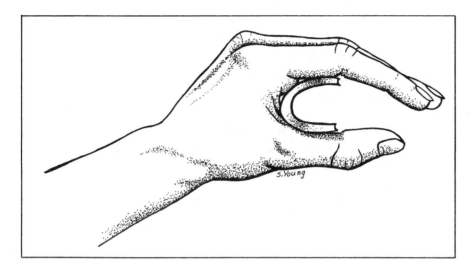

Figure 3-17. Length of a **C** *bar.*

2. Width: With the patient's MP joints in extension and thumb abducted, place the paper towel that has been cut to the correct length in position on the hand. Be sure the length is placed in position where it was measured. The radial side of the paper towel should be located about one-eighth inch radial to the second metacarpal head (index finger), as seen from the dorsal side of the hand (Fig. 3–18). The ulnar edge of the **C** bar pattern will then need to be cut off at the center of the head of the third metacarpal, as seen from the volar side of the hand (Fig. 3–18).

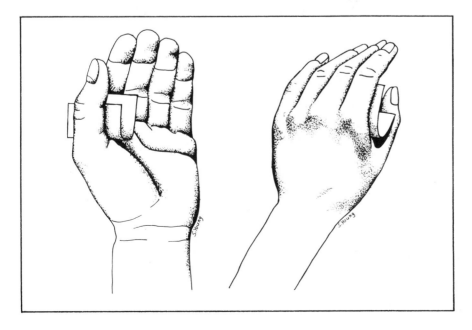

Figure 3-18. Width of a **C** *bar.*

3. At this point the **C** bar looks like a rectangle. To complete it the corners must be rounded. (A penny is useful to make uniformly rounded corners. See Fig. 3–26.) When properly formed the **C** bar is rolled or curved down (see Fig. 3–16) as much or as little as necessary for a patient. If an individual requires a very small **C** bar, the length measurements may be shortened slightly on the pattern. Care must be taken, however, that an edge that will cause pressure in the web space is not left in the splint. The length of the pattern should not be increased, and the measurements for the width of the pattern should not be altered, or the size of the pattern will become so large that it becomes a resting pan or a thumb post.

4. To attach the **C** bar pattern to the rest of the splint pattern, it is easiest to first tape both patterns to the hand before taping them together.

    a. Place the simple cock-up splint pattern on the hand in the correct position. Tape it to the hand in at least one spot at the distal end and one spot at the proximal end.

    b. Roll a small piece of tape with the sticky side out and place it in the back of the web space. Place the **C** bar in the web space in the correct position. The small roll of tape will hold it there.

    c. With both patterns taped onto the hand the ulnar edge of the **C** bar should slightly overlap, or at least come very close to, the point on the distal, radial end of the simple cock-up splint. Place a piece of tape (one-half inch wide is best) at the spot where the two pieces naturally touch (Fig. 3–19).

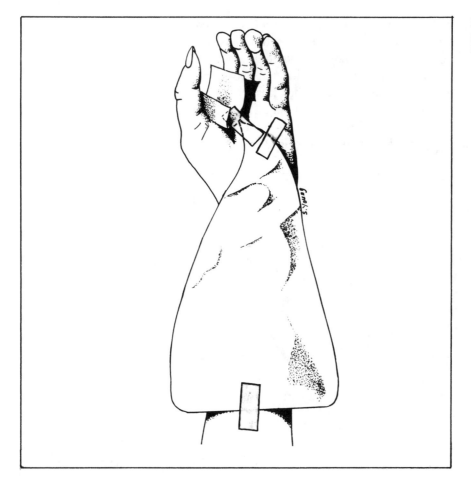

*Figure 3-19. Attaching a **C** bar pattern to a simple cock-up splint.*

5. Check the **C** bar pattern for fit.

    a. Be sure that when taped in place the **C** bar pattern adheres to the width dimensions to ensure good support of the web space and prevent the index finger from slipping off the radial edge of the splint.

    b. Check the length to ensure that it either adheres to the size described in the directions, or that it has not been shortened so much that pressure may result.

Connector Bar. The purpose of a connector bar is to position functional parts of the splint in their proper relationship on the hand.

A connector bar can be added to a pattern as necessary by cutting a small strip of paper one-half inch wide (*never* less—a large person may require more) and three to four inches long. This small strip of paper is then positioned in any small section where it is needed, to assist with the correct alignment of splint parts. An example of the use of the connector bar is in the process of attaching the opponens bar.

Opponens Bar. The purpose of an opponens bar (Fig. 3–20) is to stabilize the first metacarpal volar to the second metacarpal, so that opposition and prehension are possible.

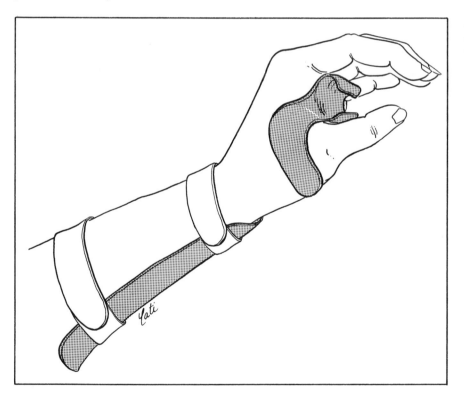

*Figure 3-20. Simple cock-up splint with **C** bar and opponens bar attachment.*

The opponens bar must be added as an attachment to the pattern of a splint. **Note:** It should be cut out as part of the same piece of plastic when making a splint, rather than adding it to the splint as an attachment. An addition of this type could be a potential source of pressure sores. If care is used, however, it can be done. Although it is possible to do without, usually when an opponens bar is added to a simple cock-up splint, a **C** bar is also added. Without a **C** bar, the connector bar may have to be widened in the web space area to prevent the development of pressure sores.

Directions for making the opponens bar pattern:

1. Cut a strip of paper about three inches long and the desired width for the completed opponens bar.

   a. In order to determine the desired width, the length of the first metacarpal must be examined to see how much width it can accommodate. Usually the width can be slightly less than one-half of the length of the first metacarpal. The width should *never* be less than one-half inch even for a very small child. (If the child is so small that one-half inch is not feasible, a different style splint should be used.) The average size woman can accommodate between five-eights and three-fourths of an inch, and a man can frequently use up to one inch width.

2. When attaching the opponens bar pattern to the rest of the splint, a connector bar is needed to position it correctly.

   a. The placement of the connector bar should be done with the **C** bar pattern in place. One end of the connector bar should be taped to the point at which the **C** bar and simple cock-up splint are attached. The remainder of the connector bar should extend through the **C** bar at the back of the web space with the excess sticking out on the radial

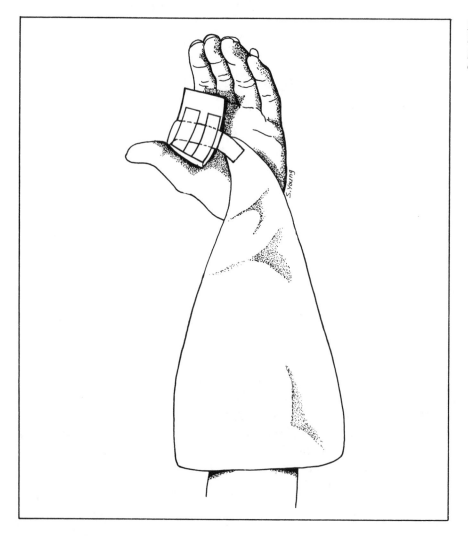

*Figure 3-21. Place a connector bar pattern over the **C** bar pattern and tape to both edges of the **C** bar.*

side of the hand. It is wise to tape the connector bar to the **C** bar on both the radial and the ulnar sides (Fig. 3–21).

b. Being careful to avoid pulling the **C** bar out of shape, pull the excess connector bar down to the surface of the skin toward the wrist, so that it lies centered between the first and second metacarpal bones (Fig. 3–22). When pulling the connector bar into place between the first and second metacarpals, be sure that the **C** bar is not pulled out of shape (Fig. 3–23). The connector bar should be the only thing to turn the corner around the hand, leaving the **C** bar to be smooth (see Fig. 3–22).

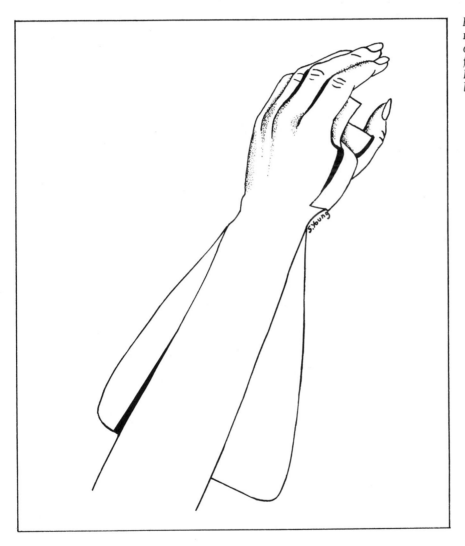

*Figure 3-22. Place the connector bar on dorsal surface of the hand between the first and second metacarpals. Do not allow it to pull the **C** bar out of shape.*

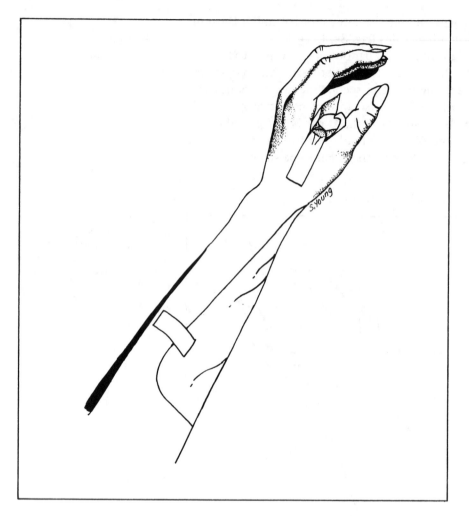

*Figure 3-23. The connector bar is pulled too tightly causing the **C** bar to be pulled out of shape.*

3. The distal and volar edges of the opponens bar pattern should be taped correctly onto the hand, making the rest of the boundaries lie correctly.

    a. The *distal* edge of the opponens bar should be placed *proximal* to the head of the first metacarpal.

    b. For length, the volar edge should be located on the surface of the skin that lies approximately in the center of the flexor pollicis brevis muscle (Fig. 3–24). In order to locate the flexor pollicis brevis the thumb should be brought across the palm with the IP held firmly in extension [1]. In this position the flexor pollicis brevis muscle can be felt and sometimes be seen. With the volar edge of the opponens bar positioned as described, it will be long enough to hold the first metacarpal opposed to the second metacarpal, but not extend onto the volar surface of the hand. When the distal and volar edges are positioned correctly, at a right angle to each other, the rest of the strip will extend dorsally and proximally from these two boundaries (Fig. 3–25).

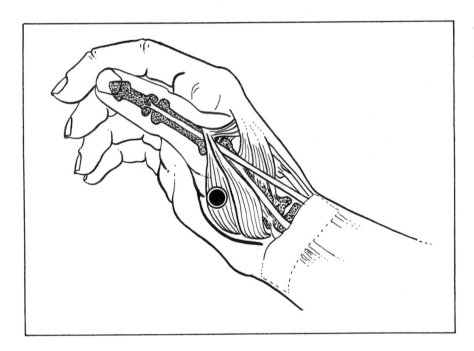

Figure 3-24. The dot indicates the center of the flexor pollicis brevis muscle.

Note: With experience it is often unnecessary to locate the flexor pollicis brevis muscle as the required length of an opponens bar becomes more familiar to the splinter.

4. With the opponens bar taped as described in 3.a and 3.b, the connector bar and opponens bar will overlap. Tape them together where they overlap naturally (Fig. 3–25). Any excess paper towel that extends dorsally or proximally to the taped overlapping area should be cut off. All corners should be rounded (Fig. 3–26).

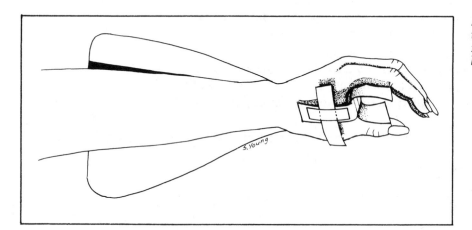

Figure 3-25. When positioned correctly the connector bar and the opponens bar overlap.

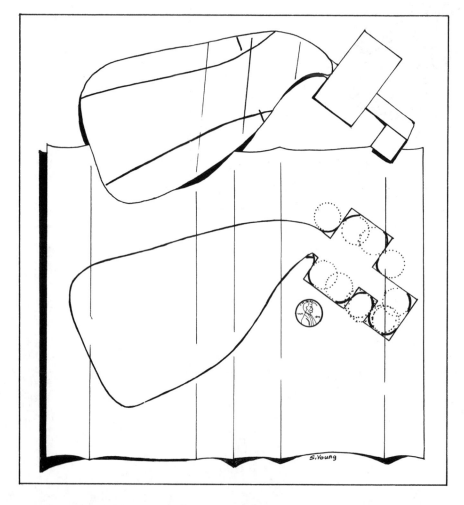

Figure 3-26. Trace the taped together pattern onto a clean paper towel and penny round all of the internal and external corners.

5. Check the opponens bar pattern for fit.

    a. Be sure that the opponens bar fits on the first metacarpal bone, proximal to the head of the metacarpal phalangeal joint, to avoid causing pressure on that joint, and to extend the length of the opponens bar lever arm as far as possible.

    b. The opponens bar should be long enough to maintain opposition, but it should not extend onto the volar surface of the hand, limiting the range of motion or obstructing sensation.

    c. The connector bar must do all the turning of the corner from the web space.

    Note: When forming the splint in plastic, the edge of a **C** bar will not bend to turn the corner.

These attachments may be added to the simple cock-up splint as needed for a patient problem. They may be used individually, in pairs, or all three. The only exception was mentioned in the discussion of the opponens bar (i.e., it is easier to fit the opponens bar and connector bar needed to attach it if there is also a **C** bar on the splint). When an opponens bar and **C** bar are added to the simple cock-up splint, they serve the purpose of a radial deviation bar for the wrist.

*Cock-up Splint with a Rolled **C** Bar*
This splint (Fig. 3–27) accomplishes the same purpose as a simple cock-up splint with a **C** bar, ulnar deviation bar, and radial deviation bar attached. With some adjustments in the way the radial side is formed, it will also function as if it had an opponens bar. Because this type of splint *must* be made from a stretchy material, none of these attachments can be removed from the splint as they can with the simple cock-up splint. The parts not only function as they were intended to function, but the splint would be

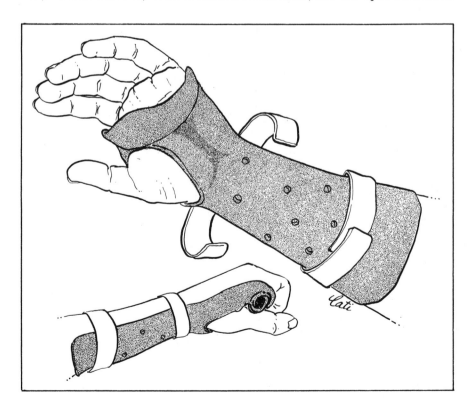

*Figure 3-27. Cock-up splint with a rolled **C** bar.*

weak, if any of the parts were eliminated. Discussion of the properties of the different plastics can be found in chapter 4. Directions for making the cock-up splint with a rolled **C** bar pattern:

1. Complete the eight steps for making a volar forearm bar pattern, pages 44–53.
2. Measure the thickness of the hand at the second MP joint and at the fifth MP joint. This can be done by having the patient place his or her hand on a flat surface and measuring vertically from the surface with a ruler. It is very likely that these two measurements will be different, the radial side being slightly larger.
   Note: With experience it becomes unnecessary to measure these distances with a ruler, as this distance can be estimated.
3. On the radial side, draw a line that extends the side of the forearm bar distal to the wrist. This will add width to the radial side of the splint in the hand area. The width added on the radial side should equal the measurement of the thickness of the second MP joint. The length of this line required distally for a rolled **C** bar depends on the size of rolled **C** bar wanted. An average place to stop for the length is adjacent to the middle phalanx of the index finger (Fig. 3–28).

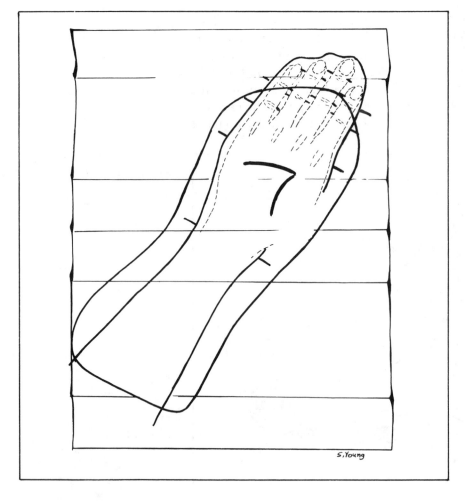

*Figure 3-28. Width and length dimensions for the pattern of a cock-up splint with a rolled **C** bar.*

4. On the ulnar side, a similar line should extend from the wrist at the ulnar side of the hand. The width added on the ulnar side should equal the measurement for the thickness of the fifth MP joint. The average length of this line is adjacent to the middle of the middle phalanx of the little finger (Fig. 3–28).

   Note: If the rolled **C** bar needed is larger or smaller than the one illustrated in Figure 3–27, the distal length lines should all be adjusted appropriately in steps 3, 4, and 5.

5. The radial and ulnar side lines should be connected with a line that goes across the fingers approximately in the center of the middle phalanges. This line should be smoothed and streamlined, however, rather than following the jagged line that would be caused by the varying lengths of the metacarpals (Fig. 3–28).

6. A hole that the thumb will go through in the splint is needed in the center of this pattern. (Because of the stretchy material used in making this splint, the size of this hole needs to be surprisingly small.) In order to properly locate the hole follow the steps below.

   a. Place a dot at the spot where the flexion crease and the thenar crease intersect. This should be located proximal to the markings for the MP joints and ulnar to the line tracing the radial side of the hand. Usually this dot is in line with the dots marking the PIPs and the DIPs between the index and middle fingers. If these guidelines are not correct, there is a problem that must be corrected before proceeding (Fig. 3–29).

   b. Sketch lines indicating the position of the forearm bones (radius and ulna) (Fig. 3–29).

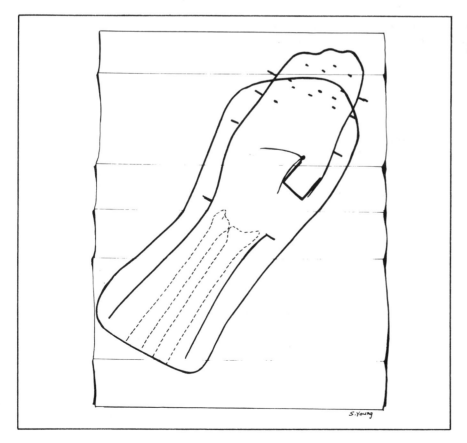

Figure 3-29. Thumb hole in pattern of cock-up splint with a rolled **C** bar.

c. Beginning at the dot made in 6.a, draw a one-inch line that is parallel to the forearm bones and extends proximally toward the wrist. *Do not* make this line longer than one inch (a child may require a shorter line.) (Fig. 3–29).

d. Beginning at the proximal end of the one-inch line drawn in 6.c, draw a second one-inch line perpendicular to the first line, going toward the radial side of the hand. *Do not* make this line longer than one inch (Fig. 3–29).

e. Beginning at the radial end of the one-inch line drawn in 6.d, draw a third one-inch line parallel to the first line and perpendicular to the second line. This line should extend distally toward the finger tips. *Do not* make this line longer than one inch. This third line completes three sides of a one-inch square; there will not be a fourth side. The third line drawn usually ends approximately in line with the radial side of the traced hand.

Note: In order for the splint to work effectively there must be three-fourths to one inch (for an adult patient) between the radial side of the thumb hole and the radial side of the splint. If this is not seen in a pattern, either the thumb hole is placed incorrectly or additional width is needed on the side of the splint (Fig. 3–29).

f. Round the two corners at the proximal end of the hole BEFORE cutting out the pattern (Fig. 3–30).

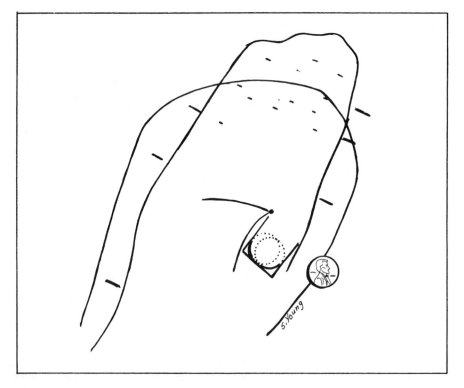

Figure 3-30. Round the corners of the thumb hole before cutting out the pattern.

Note: Earlier it was mentioned that this one-inch thumb hole size is standard and should not be enlarged, even for a very large person, because of the stretchy quality of the splinting material used. If there is a problem when fitting the splint, the thumb hole can easily be cut larger with scissors at the time the splint is formed. With children it is often necessary to decrease the size of the hole to a three-fourths or one-half inch, three-sided square.

7. Cut out the pattern, leaving the tab from the thumbhole attached. The fourth side of the square, which did not have a line drawn, must not be cut.
8. Try on the pattern for fit. Put the thumb through the hole in the center of the pattern with the tab sticking out away from the palm of the hand. Holding the hand in a functional position, check the following areas for fit.

   a. The length of the forearm should extend proximally two-thirds of the distance from the axis of the wrist joint to the elbow.
   b. The width of the forearm bar should extend just one-half the distance up each side of the forearm. This is especially important to note at the wrist, as this area can easily become too snug in the initial fitting and can make the splint painful as well as difficult to remove.
   c. The distal length is drawn between the DIP and PIP joints on the pattern; however, when measured on the hand, it will extend only to the PIP joint.
   d. The width at the MP joint should be measured by rolling the distal end of the splint two or three times until it rests at the MP joints. The width on both the radial and ulnar sides should extend around the full thickness of the radial and ulnar borders of the hand at the second and fifth MP joints. When measuring this, be sure that the pattern is held smooth and next to the palm to allow room for a transverse arch support, before looking at the width of the deviation bars. Neither of the deviation bars should extend to the dorsal surface.
   Note: If this happens, the splint will be hard to put on and take off.
   e. All corners must be rounded.

Resting Pan Splint

The purpose of a resting pan splint may be prevention of deformity (e.g., contractures from a nerve injury), immobilization of the entire hand to rest and promote healing, or protection of weak muscles from overstretching. This splint allows no motion in any joint. It holds the hand immobile in a functional position. Directions for making the resting pan splint pattern:

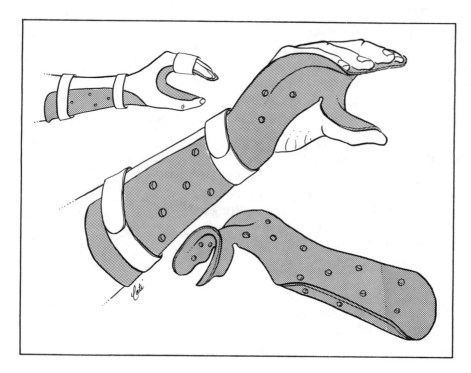

Figure 3-31. Resting pan splint.

1. Complete the eight steps for making a volar forearm bar pattern, pages 44–53.
2. Measure the thickness of the hand at the MP joints and at both IP joints of the second and fifth digits. The same procedures outlined in No. 2 for the cock-up splint with a rolled **C** bar may be used for these measurements (see page 70). Again, with experience measuring with a ruler becomes unnecessary.

3. On the radial side, draw a line that extends the side of the forearm bar distal to the wrist. This will add width to the radial side of the splint in the hand area. The width added on the radial side should be equal to the measurements taken at the second MP joint and the second PIP and DIP joints. This means that the width added should decrease slightly, and very gradually as the line moves distally. In the area of the thumb, the line should continue straight with no increase or decrease to allow for the thumb (Fig. 3–32).

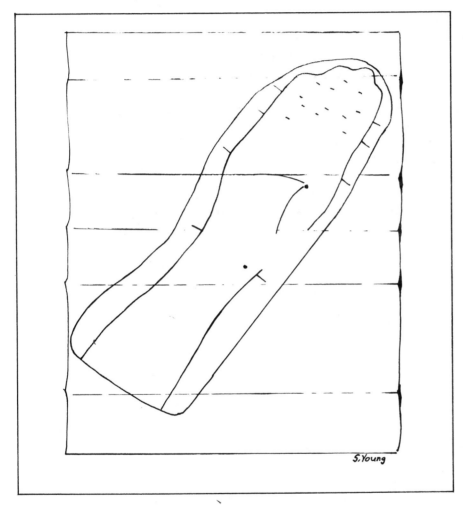

Figure 3-32. Width and length dimensions for the pattern of a resting pan splint. The dots show intersection of the flexion crease and thenar crease and the wrist.

4. The ulnar side should have a similar line extending distally from the wrist. The amount of width added on the ulnar side should equal the measurements taken at the fifth MP, PIP, and DIP joints. This will cause a gradual decrease in width as the line moves distally (Fig. 3–32).

5. To keep the splint from being unwieldly, the distal length of the pattern should not extend past the finger tips. When drawing the line for this, make it curved and smooth with its most distal point being at the tip of the third digit (Fig. 3–32).

6. Draw the thumb post onto the pattern.

   a. Place a dot at the point where the flexion crease and thenar crease intersect. See 6.a, page 71 in the directions for the cock-up splint with a rolled **C** bar for further discussion of this point (Fig. 3–32).

   b. Measure the distance between this dot and the radial side of the splint, as drawn in No. 3, page 75.

   c. At the level of the mark made for the axis of the wrist joint on the radial side, place a second dot the same distance from the edge of the splint as measured in b (Fig. 3–32).

   d. Draw a straight line, using a ruler, between the dots made in a and c. This line should be parallel to the radial side of the splint (Fig. 3–32).

   e. Draw a second line beginning at the proximal end of the first line. It should be perpendicular to the first line and stop at the radial edge of the splint (Fig. 3–33).

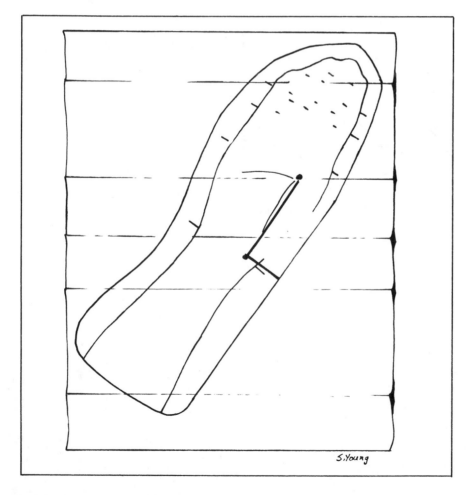

Figure 3-33. Lines marking the medial and proximal borders of the thumb post.

S. Young

f. Round the corners of the thumb post with a penny (Fig. 3–34).

g. Beginning on the first line drawn in d at the start of where the thumb post is rounded, draw another line to streamline the side of the splint as it tapers out to the radial edge of the splint. Refer to the radial edge of the simple cock-up splint pattern in the wrist area to get the idea of shape. (The purpose of this streamlining is to allow space and relieve pressure on the radial styloid process and tendons in the wrist area.) This line leaves a triangle with one curved line proximal to the wrist on the radial side. This triangle will not be part of the splint; it will be thrown away (Fig. 3–34).

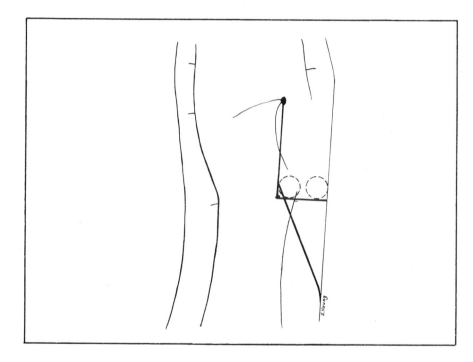

Figure 3-34. Penny round the corners of the thumb post and streamline the radial edge to avoid pressure on the radial styloid process.

7. Cut out the completed pattern, check for fit, and make any necessary adjustments (Fig. 3–35).

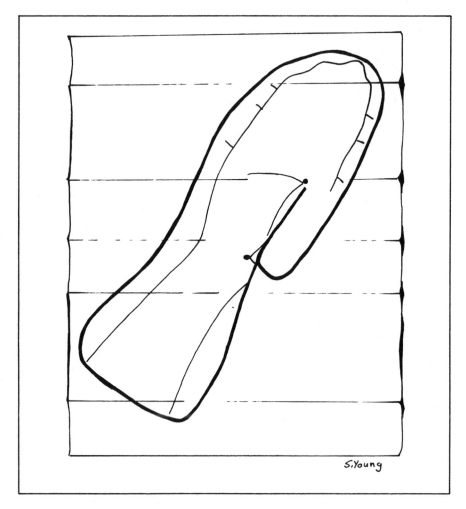

Figure 3-35. Completed pattern for a resting pan splint.

S. Young

8. When fitting this splint pattern fold or curve the thumb post toward the distal end of the splint and place the fold in the most proximal area of the web space. The areas to check for fit are:

   a. The length of the forearm should extend proximally two-thirds of the distance from the axis of the wrist joint to the elbow.

   b. The width of the forearm bar should extend just one-half of the distance up each side of the forearm. The width should not extend excessively over the ulnar or radial styloid processes in order to prevent pressure.

   c. The finger pan should extend to the tip of the fingers, but not beyond. If this length is incorrect, the thumb post should be checked to see that it was folded correctly. The fold in the thumb post is literally a pivotal point in this splint. By changing the place that this is folded, there are changes made in the length of the thumb post, the length of the finger pan, and the length of the forearm bar. The fold in the final pattern must be at the end of the cut into the splint pattern, which is the point where the flexion crease and thenar crease intersect (Fig. 3–36A and B).

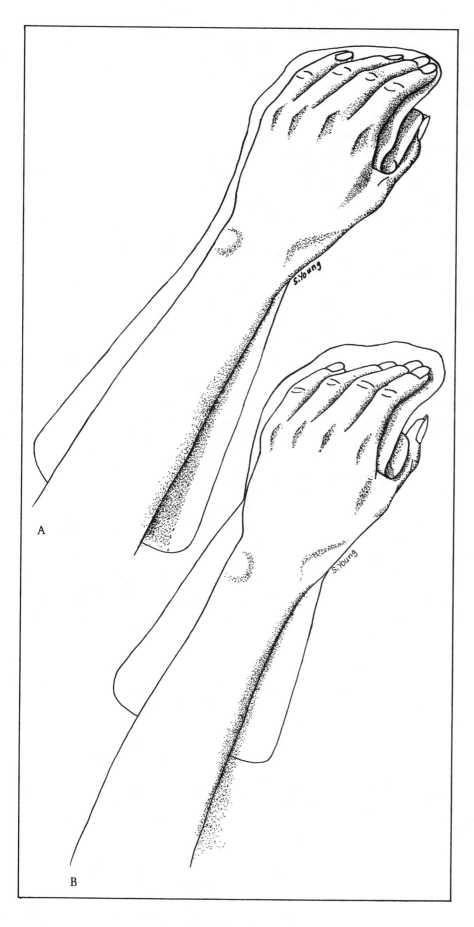

Figure 3-36. A. The pattern will fit correctly if the thumb post is folded properly. B. If the thumb post is not folded at the end of the cut, the fit of the length of the finger pan, thumb post, and forearm bar will be incorrect.

A

B

d. Finger pan width: The radial and ulnar sides of the finger pan should curve up to the level of the top of the fingers. It should not curve onto the dorsal side of the hand. There must be a small space between the fingers to allow them to rest comfortably without being crowded nor should it be so large that it does not offer any support or restraint for the fingers.

e. Thumb post length: The thumb post should not extend beyond the tip of the thumb. Usually when drawing this in the pattern, and using the axis of the wrist joint as a measuring point, the thumb post is too long, but for beginners this is a sure way to prevent having the thumb post be too short. It can be shortened easily by cutting it with scissors. When shortening the thumb post, be sure to reround the corners.

f. The thumb post should be wide enough to curve slightly around the thumb for support and to prevent deviation. This curve will also add strength to the splint. If the thumb post is not wide enough, it can be corrected by moving the entire radial edge of the splint, including the finger pan, or by moving the cut made at the thenar eminence toward the ulnar side of the splint. This decision is made based on the fit in the other areas of the splint.

Dorsal Splints

Although there are many different ways to make dorsal splints, there are two styles of palmar support seen frequently in a bar-type dorsal splint. One of these was developed at Georgia Warm Springs Foundation and is called a Warm Springs splint (Fig. 3–37). With this splint, the dorsal metacarpal bar has attachments going both to the radial and to the ulnar sides of the hand. There is a space left in the palm between the hypothenar bar and the **C** bar. This type of palmar support is referred to as indirect support. The **C** bar supports the second and third metacarpals, and the hypothenar bar supports the fourth and fifth metacarpals. The basic principle supporting this splint is that there will be more skin left open to provide sensory input to the hand.

Figure 3-37. Warm Springs long opponens splint.

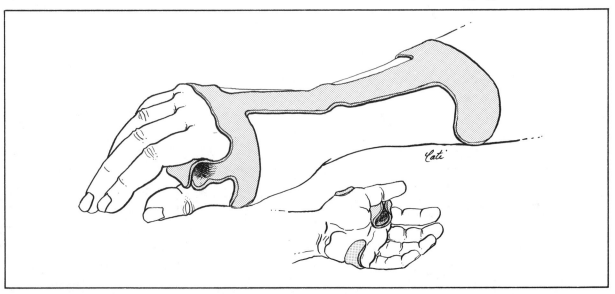

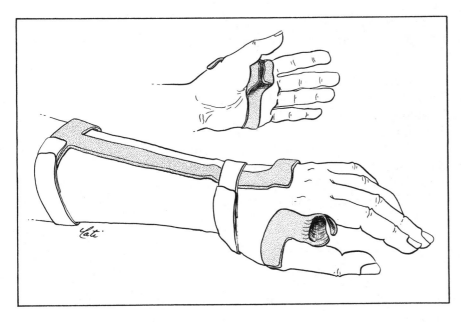

Figure 3-38. Rancho long opponens splint.

The other type of palmar arch support for a bar-type dorsal splint was developed at Rancho Los Amigos Hospital in Downey, California. The Rancho splint (Fig. 3–38) has all the attachments for the transverse arch support extending from the ulnar side of the dorsal metacarpal bar. There is what could be thought of as an extension from the hypothenar bar connecting it to the **C** bar, or it could be considered a connector bar between the two parts. The Rancho splint offers direct support to the transverse arch because there is no space left in the palm of the hand. Although this does allow less area in the palm for sensory stimulation, the arch support appears to be more effective, especially with a hand that is flaccid or extremely weak.

Bar-Type Short Opponens Splint
The purpose of this splint is to maintain the thumb in opposition so that prehension occurs. It usually has a **C** bar to maintain the web space, and it will support the transverse arch with either direct or indirect support. Directions for making a Warm Springs short opponens splint pattern:

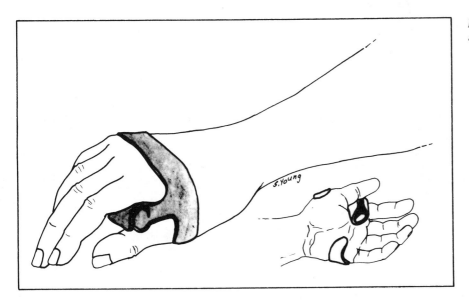

Figure 3-39. Warm Springs short opponens splint.

1. Place a strip of paper towel that has been cut to the desired width on the dorsal surface of the metacarpal bones of the hand. A positive mold of the hand may be used to make this pattern (see p. 101).

   a. The desired width must be determined for each hand that is being splinted. One way this can be determined is described in the discussion of how wide to make an opponens bar (see p. 64).

   b. This strip of paper towel should be placed with the center on top of the third metacarpal bone. The distal edge should be parallel and proximal to the third, fourth, and fifth metacarpal heads. Tape the paper towel in place proximal to the heads of these three metacarpals, leaving it loose radial to the third metacarpal and ulnar to the fifth metacarpal (Fig. 3–40).

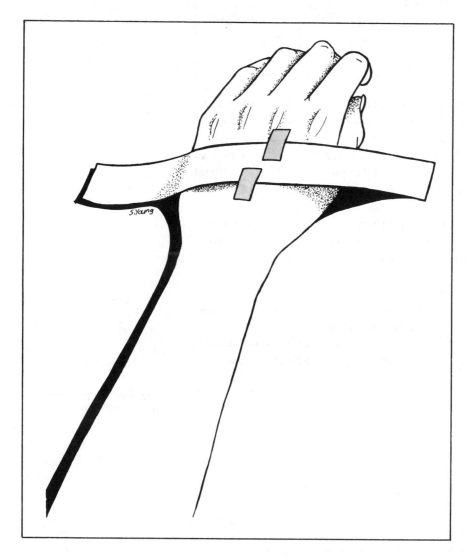

Figure 3-40. Place the center of the strip of paper towel on the dorsal surface of meta-carpals. The distal edge is parallel to the third, fourth, and fifth metacarpal heads.

2. With the hand held in a functional position, grasp the radial side of the crosswise strip, and pull it toward the wrist until the distal edge is just proximal to the first metacarpal head. This position is the distal edge of the opponens bar. (The paper towel will not be lying flat on the hand at this point.) Press a tuck into the paper towel, so that it will lie flat on the dorsum of the hand. Tape this tuck in place (Fig. 3–41). Cut off the end of this radial strip to the desired length. See pages 67 and 68 for a description of how long to make an opponens bar.

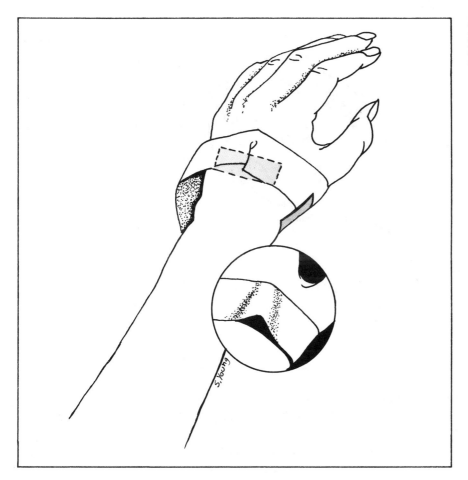

Figure 3-41. Tape a tuck in the paper towel so that it will lie flat in the correct position on the hand.

3. Grasp the ulnar side of the strip and pull it around the ulnar side of the hand to the volar surface, to make a hypothenar bar. Place the distal edge of this strip on the flexion crease in the palm of the hand. The paper towel on the ulnar side of the hand should not be lying flat. Press a second tuck into the paper towel to make it lie flat, then tape it in place (Fig. 3–42).
4. Cut off the end of this hypothenar bar to end in the middle of the fourth metacarpal on the volar surface of the hand. See Fig. 3–39, which shows where the splint should extend in the palm of the hand.
5. Make a pattern for a **C** bar (see pp. 60–63).

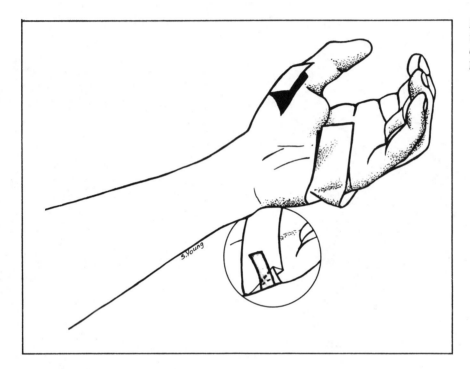

Figure 3-42. Tape a tuck on the ulnar side to place the distal edge in line with the flexion crease.

6. Make a pattern for a connector bar and attach it to the **C** bar and opponens bar (see p. 63). Cut off any excess connector bar that extends proximal to the opponens bar.
7. Remove taped-together pattern from the hand or positive mold, and trace it onto a new paper towel. Straighten or smooth the edges as appropriate, and penny round all corners.
8. Fit the traced pattern onto the *hand*, being sure all parts fit as originally measured.

Directions for making a Rancho short opponens splint pattern:

1. Place a strip of paper towel that has been cut to the desired width on the dorsal surface of the metacarpal bones of the hand. A positive mold of the hand may be used to make this pattern (see p. 101). One way to determine the desired width for this splint is to follow the directions for determining the desired width of the opponens bar (see p. 64).

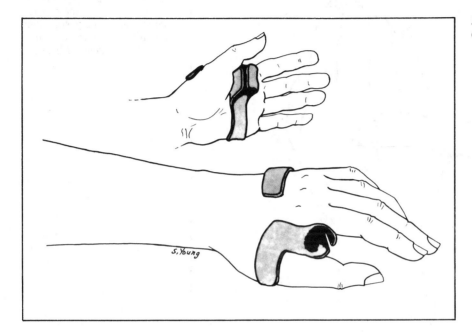

Figure 3-43. Rancho short opponens splint.

a. This strip of paper towel should be placed with the radial end on top of the third metacarpal bone. The distal edge should be parallel and proximal to the third, fourth, and fifth metacarpal heads. Tape the paper towel in place proximal to these three metacarpal heads, leaving it loose ulnar to the fifth metacarpal (Fig. 3–44).

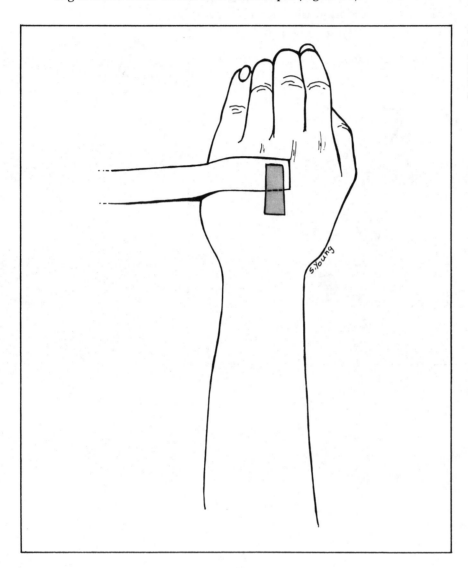

Figure 3-44. Place the radial end of the strip of paper towel on the dorsal surface of the metacarpals. The distal edge is parallel to the third, fourth, and fifth metacarpal heads.

2. Grasp the ulnar side of the strip and pull it around the ulnar side of the hand to the volar surface to make a hypothenar bar. Place the distal edge of this strip on the flexion crease in the palm of the hand. The towel on the ulnar side of the hand will not be lying flat. Press a tuck into the paper towel to make it lie flat, then tape it in place. See Figure 3–42, page 84 for the correct placement of the hypothenar bar and how to tape the tuck. Allow the remainder of the strip of paper towel to go through the most proximal part of the web space.

3. Using the directions for a **C** bar (see pp. 60–63) and the directions for an opponens bar (see pp. 63–69), add these attachments to the pattern. The remainder of the original strip of paper towel that is extending through the web space can be used for the connector bar. Be sure when attaching the **C** bar that it lies next to the skin and that the connector bar is placed on top of it. This will help ensure that the connector bar is used to go around the corner of the hand rather than the **C** bar being pulled out of shape.

4. Remove the taped-together pattern from the hand or positive mold, and trace it onto a new paper towel. Straighten or smooth the edges, as appropriate, and penny round all corners.

5. Fit the traced pattern on the *hand*, being sure all parts fit as originally measured.

Bar-Type Long Opponens Splint. If either of the above short opponens splints are desired, but the wrist needs to be stabilized, a forearm bar may be added to the pattern before the original is traced. Directions for a bar type dorsal forearm bar follow. These directions may be used for either a Rancho or Warm Springs splint (see Figs. 3–37, 3–38).

1. Tape one pencil across the dorsal surface of the wrist so that the end on the ulnar side goes over the ulnar styloid process. Again, the use of a positive mold of the hand may be desirable (Fig. 3–45).

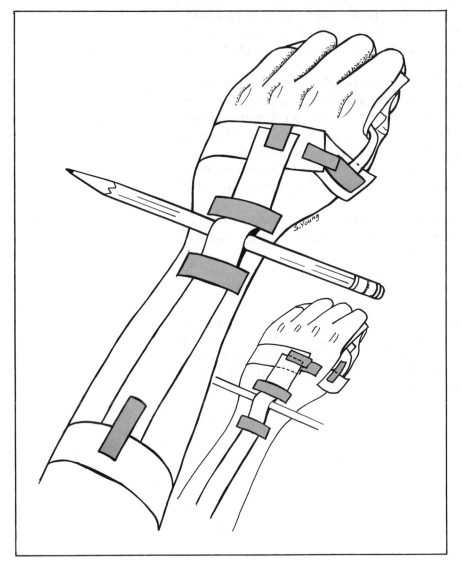

Figure 3-45. Attachment of a dorsal forearm bar to a short opponens splint. A pencil is positioned over the ulnar styloid process to ensure that enough plastic is provided in the forearm bar to avoid pressure on the styloid process.

2. Using the same width strip of paper towel that has been used for the rest of the splint, place a strip of paper towel on the center of the dorsal surface of the forearm. The distal end should be located on top of the third metacarpal and taped to the paper towel that is located across the metacarpals of the hand. None of this strip of paper towel should extend distal to the original strip of paper towel (Fig. 3–45).
3. Tape this strip of paper towel to the skin on both sides of the pencil, forming a hump in the splinting pattern. This will allow a hump to be placed in the forearm bar of the plastic splint, which will help prevent pressure on the ulnar styloid process (Fig. 3–45).
4. The proximal end of this strip of paper towel should be cut off at a point that is two-thirds of the distance from the axis of the wrist joint to the elbow flexion crease. See page 47 for further discussion of the length of a forearm bar.

5. Place a cross bar at the end of, and perpendicular to, the dorsal forearm bar. The cross bar should be the same width as the rest of the splint and should extend about halfway around the forearm. The placement of the cross bar must not lengthen the forearm bar.
6. Remove the taped-together pattern from the hand or positive mold, and trace it onto a new paper towel. Straighten or smooth the edges, as appropriate, and penny round all corners.
7. Fit the traced pattern on the *hand*, being sure all parts fit as originally measured.

Lumbrical Bar. If hyperextension of the metacarpal phalangeal joints is a problem, a lumbrical bar may be needed. To prevent pressure on the dorsal surface of the metacarpal bones, the use of a forearm bar is recommended to be used with a lumbrical bar that covers all four fingers. The following directions for making a pattern for a lumbrical bar may be used for either a Rancho or Warm Springs splint (Fig. 3–46).

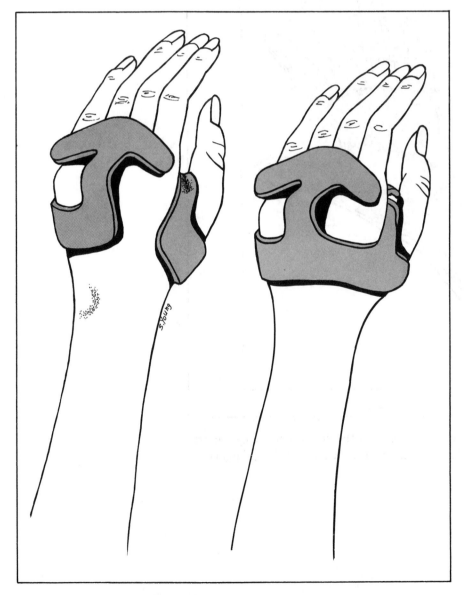

Figure 3-46. A lumbrical bar attached to a Rancho (left) or a Warm Springs (right) short opponens splint.

1. Trace around hand and all fingers on a paper towel. Fingers should be spread about three-fourths to one inch apart at the distal end.
2. Mark as deeply as possible in the web spaces between all fingers.
3. Mark both sides of the axis of all the interphalangeal joints and the axis of the second and fifth metacarpal phalangeal joints.
4. Remove the hand from the paper towel. The lumbrical bar fits between the metacarpal phalangeal joints and the proximal interphalangeal joints. Draw a line inside these two boundaries and extend the line beyond the outside borders of the second and fifth fingers about one-quarter inch (slightly more or less if the hand is very large or very small). The width of the lumbrical bar is usually not uniform, as it must be as wide as possible but still not cause pressure on any of the eight joints that surround it (Fig. 3–47).

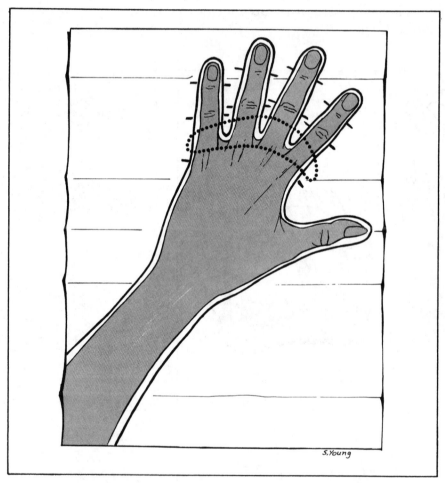

Figure 3-47. Making a lumbrical bar pattern.

5. Cut out the lumbrical bar and place it on the dorsal surface of the first phalanx of the fingers. Be sure that the lines that traced the fingers are lined up correctly.

6. After being cut out and placed on the hand one/or both of the ends (radial or ulnar) of the lumbrical bar may seem to be too far proximal and cover some of the metacarpal phalangeal joint. If this occurs, move the proximal edge into a desired position distal to the MP joint and tape a tuck in the lumbrical bar to maintain the correct shape (Fig. 3–48). Set the correctly shaped lumbrical bar aside.

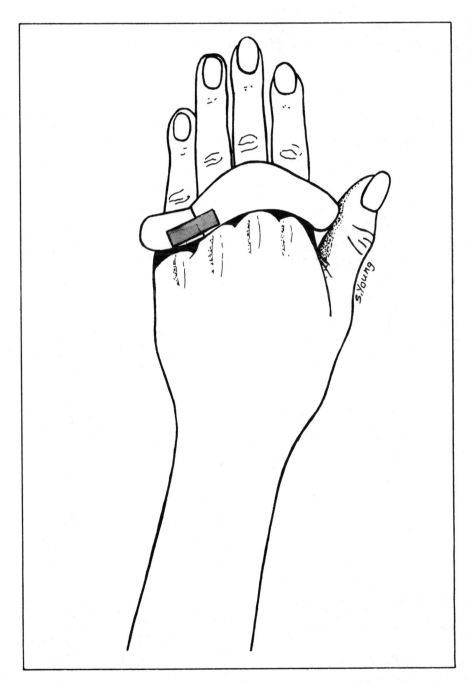

Figure 3-48. A tuck may have to be taped on the ulnar end of the lumbrical bar to prevent pressure on the fifth metacarpal head.

7. Tape a pencil to the dorsal surface of the third metacarpal phalangeal joint so that it lies perpendicular to the third metacarpal bone.

8. Using the same width strip of paper towel that has been used for the rest of the splint, place a strip of paper towel over the third metacarpal phalangeal joint and the pencil that is taped over it. The strip of paper towel will be a connector bar. It should be taped to the paper towel that is located across the metacarpals of the hand, with none of it extending proximal to the original splint pattern for the short opponens splint. The distal end of this paper towel should end in the middle of the proximal phalanx of the third digit (Fig. 3–49).

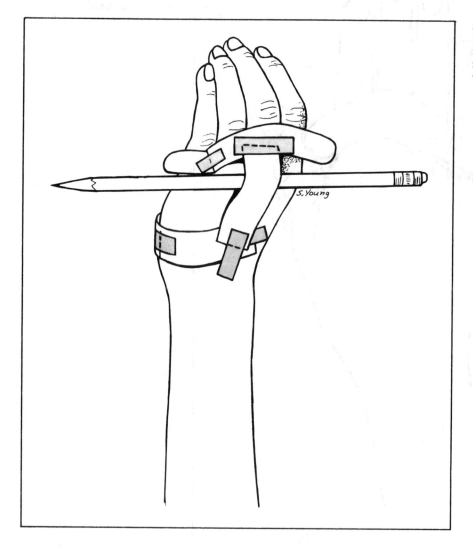

Figure 3-49. A pencil placed under the pattern will ensure that there is enough space for the metacarpals to flex without pressure.

9. Tape the lumbrical bar in the proper position on the connector bar (Fig. 3–49).

10. Remove the taped-together pattern from the hand or positive mold, and trace it onto a new paper towel. Straighten or smooth the edges as appropriate, and penny round all corners. Use caution when straightening or smoothing the edges of the lumbrical bar as it would be very easy to smooth curves that are necessary to avoid pressure on a joint.

11. Fit the traced pattern onto the *hand*, being sure all parts fit as originally measured.

The newer low temperature plastics (see Chap. 4) have done a great deal to simplify the process of making splints. Bar-type splints, like those just described, are frequently bypassed in favor of a design that has more curving contour and will permit the use of low temperature plastics. A wide dorsal forearm bar can be made in a size and shape similar to a volar forearm bar. When a narrow bar is necessary, a hollow or solid tube of low temperature plastic is used, and the tube shape has the necessary contour for strength. Another option for a narrow bar is the use of some type of strong wire that is attached to the base splint.

The principles of fit that are found in the patterns in this book all apply with only occasional modification when using low temperature plastics. A novice splinter will find it advantageous to follow these detailed directions at the start, to learn where each part is supposed to fit, and then begin working with adaptations.

Many experienced therapists are able to cut out a general shape without a strict pattern and mold it on the patient's arm, trimming and folding where necessary. With some of the plastics it is also possible to stick on an attachment and rub the edges completely smooth. This technique does not cause pressure or poor aesthetic quality. However, since this book is intended for the novice, these techniques have been excluded. The experienced therapist who employs these techniques usually is so comfortable with splinting that specific details are automatically included, sometimes without the therapist being consciously aware of them.

Negative and Positive Molds

It is sometimes helpful to have a mold of the patient's hand when making splints. This mold can be used to make a pattern for the splint, and sometimes to begin forming the splint. It usually cannot be used to complete the splint, however. The patient's hand should be used for the final fitting of the splint. Figure 3–50 shows a positive mold and a negative mold from which the positive mold is made. A positive mold should be made for any of the following reasons.

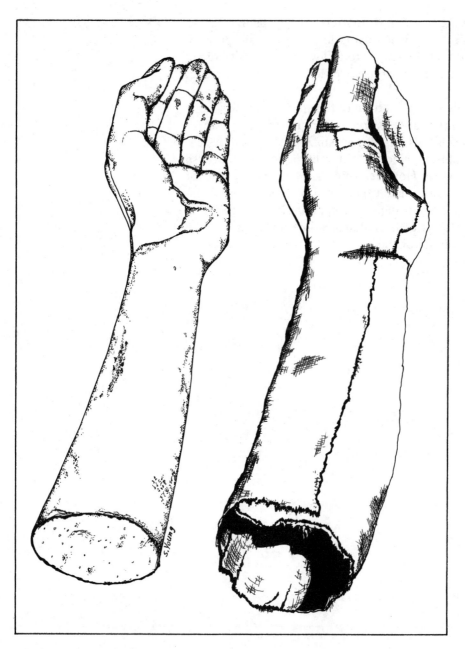

Figure 3-50. A positive mold of the hand (left) has been made from the negative mold of the hand (right).

1. The patient who will not hold still.
2. The problem is unusual or difficult and too time-consuming for the patient to be present for designing and beginning the splint.
3. A plastic that has a high forming temperature is being used.
4. The therapist or the patient does not have time to work on the splint immediately.

In order to make a positive mold, a negative mold is necessary first; then the positive mold is made from it (Fig. 3–50).

A negative mold is a hollow shell of plaster-impregnated bandage that has been formed over a particular object. Its purpose is to allow a duplicate of the object to be made by filling the mold with a liquid plaster. When the liquid plaster hardens, the negative mold is stripped away. The duplicate object is then referred to as a positive mold (Fig. 3–50).

A total of about one hour working time is needed for the completion of a negative and a positive mold. This is not necessarily one solid hour, but can be thirty minutes initially followed by two fifteen minute periods later. Thirty minutes is usually sufficient to form the negative, remove it from the patient, and patch it together in the correct shape. Fifteen minutes is needed to mix the plaster of Paris, pour it into the negative, and get it hard enough to lie down. The last fifteen minutes *must* be at least two hours later to peel the negative off the positive and prepare the positive for use.

Making a Negative Mold
Tools needed for a negative mold are these:

Pan of warm water
Bandage scissors
Vaseline or similar lubricant
Two rolls of 3-inch wide plaster bandage
Apron, smock, or gown to protect the patient's and the therapist's clothes
Newspaper

Procedure for making a negative mold is as follows.

1. Cover working area with newspaper; this job is messy.
2. Cut several lengths and sizes from the plaster bandages. You will need six to eight strips long enough to reach down either side of the forearm and over the fingertips and four strips approximately eight inches long, cut to half width.
3. Position the patient at a corner of the table so that the arm is accessible from several angles. Then place the plaster farthest from the corner on which you are working, with the water in the middle, and the patient's arm near the edge of the table. This will prevent your dripping water on the dry plaster bandage, which would ruin it (Fig. 3–51).

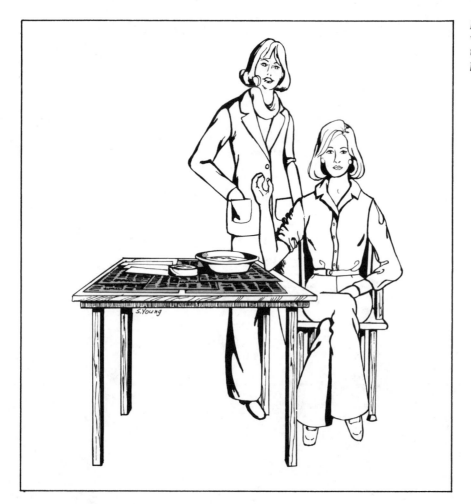

Figure 3-51. Position the water closest to the patient to avoid dripping on the dry plaster.

4. Thoroughly cover the patient's arm and hand with Vaseline. Put an extra amount over the hair covered areas and stroke the hair in the direction that it grows so that it will lie down.

5. Have the patient hold his or her hand in a functional position. Do not allow the fingers to be overly flexed, as this makes it difficult to remove the positive mold from the negative mold. If the patient is unable to maintain the position, have an assistant help hold or use masking tape to help position the hand.

6. Fold (do not wad) a long strip of plaster loosely into your hand; dip it into the water for about five seconds. Squeeze it gently, being careful not to wash out all of the plaster (Fig. 3–52).

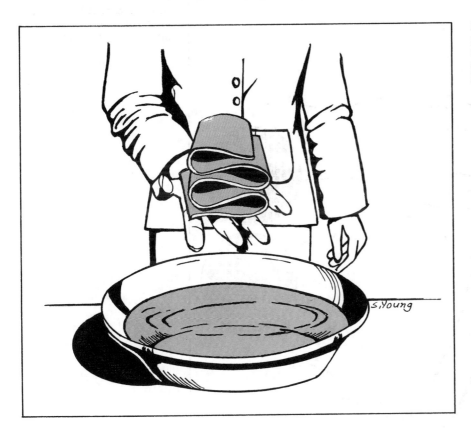

Figure 3-52. Carefully fold the plaster bandage to dip it into the water. Avoid washing all of the plaster out of the bandage.

7. Apply the strip down the midline of the patient's forearm and over the
   fingers. Apply the next strip on the opposite side and over the finger.
   Note: It is sometimes easier, when molding a negative over a flaccid
   hand, to put plaster on just part of the hand at one time. In this way the
   plaster covering the wrist can harden before attempting to position
   the fingers. Position the thumb last (Fig. 3–53).

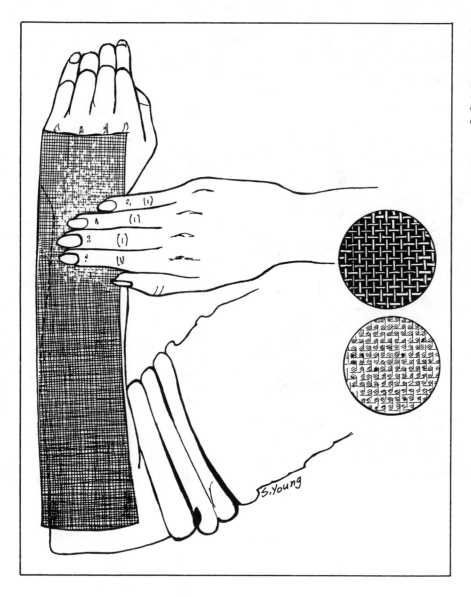

*Figure 3-53. Rub the wet
plaster into all of the pores of
the bandage. The circle at the
top indicates the appearance
prior to rubbing the plaster
into the bandage. The circle
at the bottom indicates the
appearance after rubbing.*

8. Smooth the plaster bandage on the patient's skin, snip it as necessary to avoid wrinkles, and fit it into all skin creases (Fig. 3–54).

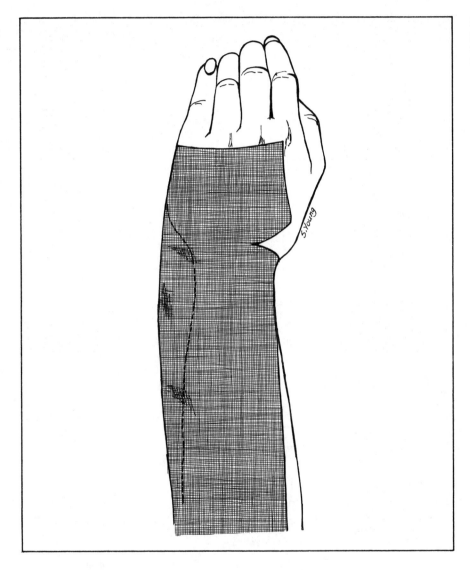

Figure 3-54. Clip the wet plaster bandage with scissors to help it lay smoothly on the arm.

9. Overlay additional strips on both sides of the first and second strips. Smooth as before until the weave of the cloth is thoroughly filled with plaster and no holes are visible. Two or three thicknesses of plaster bandage are sufficient; *do not get the negative too thick* or it will be very difficult to remove from the patient's arm.

10. Use the narrow pieces to wrap the thumb and finger tips. Be sure to attach them firmly to the rest of the hand mold.

11. Reinforce the thumb web area with small pieces of plaster bandage.

12. Wrap an additional strip of plaster bandage around the forearm at right angles to the previous strips.

13. Allow the plaster to set for about five minutes or until it has had time to become hard.

14. Ask the patient to pronate and supinate his or her forearm to help loosen the mold.

15. With bandage scissors (blunt tip next to the skin) cut the mold down the radial side of the forearm. In order to plan as well as to reassure the patient, it may be helpful to draw a line on the mold where you plan to cut it (Fig. 3–55).

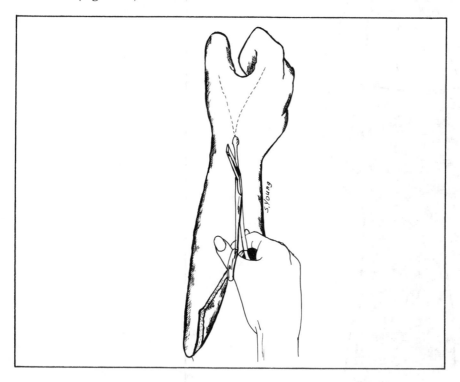

Figure 3-55. The negative mold is cut down the radial side in order to remove it from the arm.

16. Be cautious when cutting the mold in the wrist area as it is most likely to hurt the patient in this area.

17. End the cut in a **Y** shape following the radial aspect of the first and second metacarpals. Do not attempt to cut across the top of the heads of the metacarpals, but cut beside them and stop just distal to them.

18. Carefully slide the patient's hand out of the mold (Fig. 3–56).

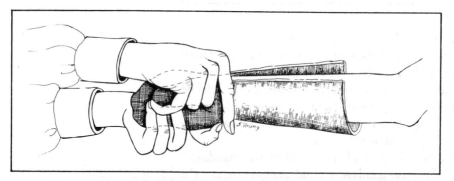

Figure 3-56. Carefully support the fingers and thumb when removing the negative mold from the patient's arm.

19. Patch the cut in the negative mold with plaster strips from the outside to close all cuts and reinforce the thin areas in the mold. Thin areas can be located by holding the mold up to a light source and looking inside the mold for areas that the light shines through. A dowel rod or something else that is long and skinny can be used to help smooth rough areas inside the mold that cannot be reached with a hand.

Making a Positive Mold
Tools needed for a positive mold are these:

Pencil or felt tipped pen
Plaster of Paris
Water
Pan for mixing plaster
Separator (one part liquid soap, one part kerosene, and one part water)

Procedure for making a positive mold is as follows.

1. Quickly coat the inside of the negative mold with separator. Make sure all areas are coated. It is easiest to pour the separator into the mold, swirl it around, and then pour it out again. If the mold is turned as the separator is poured out, the entire inside should be coated. Be sure to pour the separator out of the mold as quickly as possible as the liquid could cause the negative mold to collapse if it is left in too long (Fig. 3–57).

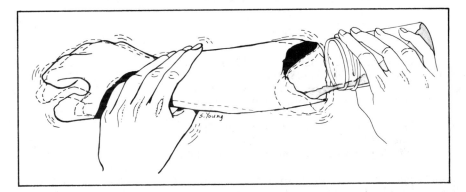

Figure 3-57. Quickly coat the inside of the negative mold with separator.

2. Mix plaster into a quart of water until it is the consistency of thick cream. Stir it with your hands to get rid of the lumps.
3. Pour the plaster into the negative mold immediately. In order to be sure that the fingers are filled completely, pour a small amount of the plaster down the side of the mold, then shake it to cause it to settle into the fingers. Proceed to fill the rest of the mold with plaster (Fig. 3–58).

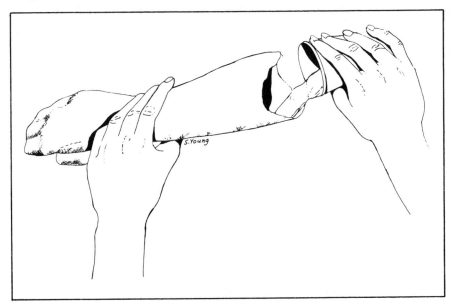

Figure 3-58. Pour the plaster down the radial side and be sure the thumb and fingers are filled before filling the forearm with plaster.

4. Hold the mold in a vertical position until it begins to harden. It can then be laid down to complete the hardening process.

5. Let the plaster harden until it is cooling again after the warm stage. About two hours is a sufficient length of time to wait. It is important that the negative be peeled off of the positive within 24 hours, as it becomes much more difficult to remove as time passes.

6. With your fingers tear away the negative mold; be especially careful in the thumb area as it can fracture easily there. Scissors or an X-Acto knife may be helpful when peeling off the negative.

7. Be sure to label the positive with the patient's name either in the wet plaster before it is entirely hardened, or on the dry plaster with a felt tipped pen.

References

1. Wynn Parry, C. B. *Rehabilitation of the Hand* (3rd ed.). London: Butterworth, 1973.

Suggested Reading

Anderson, M. H. *Upper Extremity Orthotics.* Springfield, Ill.: Thomas, 1965.

Capener, N. The hand in surgery. *J. Bone Joint Surg.* 38B(1):128, 1956.

Carl, T. K. B. Unpublished data, 1971. Revised by M. E. Fess, and J. H. Kiel, 1973.

Farber, S. D. *Neurorehabilitation: A Multisensory Approach.* Philadelphia: Saunders, 1982.

Institute and Workshop on Hand Splinting Construction. Pittsburgh: Harmarville Rehabilitation Center, March 9–11, June 2, 1967.

Malick, M. H. *Manual on Static Hand Splinting* (2nd ed.). Pittsburgh: Harmarville Rehabilitation Center, 1972.

Moore, J. C. *Adaptive Equipment and Appliances.* Ann Arbor: Overbeck, 1962.

Nickel, V. L., Perry, J., and Snelson, R. *Handbook of Handsplints.* Downey, Calif.: Rancho Los Amigos Hospital.

O'Connor, J. R. Medical Aspects of Splinting. In E. R. Mayerson (Ed.), *Splinting Theory and Fabrication.* Clarence Center, N.Y.: Goodrich, 1971.

4. Splinting Materials

There have been many different materials used for making splints throughout the years. These include plaster of Paris bandages, aluminum, fiberglass, Celastic, Lexon, Merlon, and others. All of these work with varying degrees of success, and each has its advantages and disadvantages. Today, however, there are several new plastics and some older plastics that have become quite popular as splinting materials. None of these is as durable as aluminum or as inexpensive as plaster of Paris bandages, but when considering cosmesis of the splint, ease and speed of construction, and wear and tear on the therapist, the plastics come out ahead almost every time.

The plastic materials that have been included in this text have certain characteristics the therapist should have knowledge of in order to make the effectiveness of the splint much greater. Following is a discussion of these characteristics. See Table 3, pages 105–107 for the characteristics of specific plastics.

Thermoplasticity

The plastics on the market that are currently used for splinting all have a characteristic called thermoplasticity. This means that the materials will become moldable when heat is applied and will resume their rigid state when cooled. This quality allows the therapist to heat the plastic, hold it in a desired shape during the time that it cools, and then have a rigid splint in the necessary position. If an error is made, or if the patient's needs change after a period of time, the thermoplastic quality remains. This allows the material to be reheated, remolded, and recooled several times. Theoretically there is no limit to the number of times a material can be remolded in this manner. In practice, however, it has been found that after many remoldings some of the materials, especially those with lower forming temperatures and the ability to stretch, lose some of their strength and become less aesthetically appealing.

Elastic Memory

Elastic memory is another characteristic present in some of the plastics. This characteristic causes a piece of plastic that has been formed to return to its original shape (flat) when it is reheated. Plastics without elastic memory, when heated, will drape with gravity's pull and collapse into a lump if not prevented from doing so. Plastics without elastic memory are relatively new to the market of splinting supplies. Even more recent are materials with only a small amount of the ingredient that causes elastic memory. This newest chemical makeup allows the therapist to have a bit of the best of both worlds.

It is necessary to take four precautions that are caused by the presence of thermoplasticity and possibly elastic memory.

1. Warn the patient to wash the splint only in *cold* water.
2. Avoid leaving the splint in a hot, sunny place.
3. Be sure that the parts that have been molded are completely cool before reheating an area. Cooling these parts will keep the heat from diffusing across the splint, causing the loss of some desired shape that has been molded.

4. When heating a section of the splint after another section has been molded, care must be taken not to reheat the completed area, causing it to lose its shape.

Heat Sources

There are two general types of heat source that can be used when splinting: wet and dry. Wet heat is hot water that is heated in an electric skillet, an Aquapan (especially designed for splinting), a pan on a stove or hot plate, a hydroculator, or, in some cases, tap water. Dry heat is hot air that is heated by means of a dry electric skillet, an oven, an *electric* stove burner, a heat lamp used in a protected area, or a heat gun. *Never use an open flame.*

If a wet or dry electric skillet, an oven, or anything that heats the entire splint is used, it is necessary to have a second heat source that can heat just a small area of the splint, in order to make necessary corrections without losing the shape of areas that have been formed correctly. Most therapists prefer a heat gun for this step. It is possible to make splints using only one heat source, but it is frequently not as easy.

It is necessary, while forming splints with hot plastic, to protect the therapist's hands, as well as the patient being splinted. Canvas work gloves or stockinette or both can be used for this purpose. A layer or two of stockinette covering the patient's arm is often sufficient and does not significantly change the size of the arm, although it may leave an impression in some of the softer plastics. With some of the newer splinting materials that have lower forming temperatures, it may not be necessary to cover the skin to protect it from the heat. If this is attempted, care must be used in timing the application of the plastic to the patient's skin. Note the sensitivity of the patient to heat and inform the patient that the plastic will feel warm. Special care must be observed when splinting patients who have skin that is hypersensitive to heat or who have decreased sensation.

Tracing the Pattern onto the Plastic

When tracing a pattern onto the plastic, use an implement that will mark the material clearly for cutting purposes, but preferably one that will not leave permanent marks. If the tracing marks cannot be washed off, be sure that they are cut into the waste plastic when cutting out the splint.

The table that follows is an attempt to present several of the best plastics currently used for splinting. Because manufacturers continue to improve their products, and new products are introduced, it is important for the therapist to keep abreast of the current trends. A beginning therapist should learn the basic techniques and become adept with one or two materials, then branch out to new materials as they become available, improving technique while experimenting with these [1].

Table 3. *Plastics Currently Available for Splinting*

Characteristics	Kydex [5]	Bioplastic B and BX [2]	Royalite [2]
Color	Variety	Translucent blue-gray	Variety
Manufacturer	Rohm and Haas	American Hoechst	Uniroyal Plastic Products
Types of splints	(1) Splints requiring *no* stretch, (2) splints having little curving contour, (3) bar-type splints, (4) splints for heavy or active people, including children		
Drawing device	Lead pencil Water soluble felt-tip pen	Grease pencil China marking pencil	Lead pencil Water soluble felt-tip pen
Cutting out splints and finishing edges	These materials must be cut out with a band saw, jig saw, or sabre saw. The edges must be finished first by using a belt sander or hand file to remove the large, very coarse pieces of plastic left on the edge by the saw. Sandpaper will remove the small scratches that remain. The results of using sandpaper should leave nothing that could catch a fingernail used in inspecting the edge. Medium grade steel wool should then be used to buff the edge and leave it as smooth and shiny as the face of the plastic. Steel wool can also be used on the face of Bioplastic to mask any small scratches that appear on the surface.		
Procedure for use	(1) Trace the pattern for the splint onto the plastic using the appropriate drawing device. (2) Cut out the splint shape with a saw. (3) Finish all of the edges of the splint with a file, sandpaper, and steel wool. Heat and mold the splint. Because these materials do have a higher forming temperature, it may be desirable to begin fitting the splint on a positive mold. If the patient's arm is going to be used, 2 or 3 layers of stockinette should be used to protect the arm. In addition, the splint should not be left in contact with the arm any longer than is necessary to determine what position to hold the plastic in while it cools.		
Forming temperature	200–225°F (93–107°C)	180–200°F (82–93°C)	200–225°F (93–107°C)
Recommended type of heat	Dry heat: A heat gun may be used to make the entire splint, or the whole piece of plastic may be heated using an oven or dry electric skillet. The heat gun or an electric stove burner must then be used to heat smaller areas and make necessary changes.		
Tendency to adhere	None	None	None
Working characteristics	These are very rigid and strong materials with a great deal of elastic memory. All of the materials have 1–3 min. working time, but excessive heat is felt for some time after the plastic is rigid. *Note:* Kydex and Royalite have one smooth surface and one textured surface. Some texts advocate placing either the smooth or the textured surface next to the patient's skin for various reasons. The author believes that it does not make any difference which side is placed next to the skin as long as all parts of the splint have the same side placed away from the arm. *Note:* There is a plastimer in this material that makes it difficult to break. The plastimer becomes evident as a white discoloration in the plastic when it is placed under stress. The discoloration can be eliminated by heating the area to reduce stress. The appearance of the white discoloration indicates one of two things: (1) the material has not been heated sufficiently to form the splint, (2) the splint must have more contour added in that area in order to withstand the pressure exerted there. *Note:* Royalite has a tendency to shrink slightly when heated. This shrinkage must be allowed for when making a pattern to be used with Royalite.		

Table 3. (Continued)

Characteristics	Orthoplast [3]	San-Splint [4]	Polyform [6]
Color	White	Flesh	White
Manufacturer	Johnson and Johnson	Smith and Nephew Ltd.	Rolyan Medical Products
Types of splints	(1) Splints with a great deal of curving contour, (2) splints that require a stretchy material, (3) splints with a large surface area, (4) splints for burn patients. *Note:* The degree of rigidity in these materials mandates that care be exercised when making splints with a narrow area in a spot that receives stress. A splint made of narrow bars only should not be made from these materials.		
Drawing device	Lead pencil Scratch awl or nail	Lead pencil Scratch awl or nail	Pen Scratch awl or nail
Cutting out splints and finishing edges	Because of low forming temperatures, it is impossible to sand or buff the edges of splints made from these plastics. The friction causes heat, which softens the plastic and the rubbing (as in sanding) will make the edges rougher instead of smoother. It is necessary, therefore, to cut the edges very smoothly with scissors or roll the edges down a very small distance to remove any roughness from the vicinity of the skin.		
Procedure for use	(1) *Be sure the working area is clean.* These materials have a relatively soft surface that picks up dirt. The dirt will detract from the aesthetic quality of the splint and make it difficult or impossible for the plastic to adhere to itself, as well as increase the chances for infection in an open wound. (2) Trace the pattern for the splint onto the plastic using the appropriate drawing device. (3) Heat the entire piece of plastic. (4) Cut out the splint carefully with scissors using long smooth strokes, leaving the edges as smooth as possible. Care must be exercised to prevent the hot plastic from accidentally touching itself and adhering to itself in an undesirable spot. (5) Protect the patient's arm if necessary. (6) Reheat the cut out splint and form it. Make any necessary adjustments for fit.		
Forming temperature	160–170°F (72–77°C) Softens gradually as temperature rises.	175°F (80°C) Softens gradually as temperature rises.	150–160°F (65–72°F) These materials remain firm to 150°F, then become immediately moldable. The approximate heating time is 45 sec. If overheated there will be molding problems caused by excess stretching.
Recommended type of heat	Wet heat can be used effectively, and is often preferable, with these materials. A heat gun or other source of dry heat is often desirable to change small areas of the splint that must be adjusted. *Note:* Orthoplast and San-Splint are the only two of these materials that can be heated in a dry electric skillet or an oven when heating the entire splint. If this procedure is used, some type of carrier sheet should be used to prevent sagging and adherence to hot surfaces.		
Tendency to adhere	Will adhere when very clean, hot, and dry. This material will not stick when wet. To enhance the sticking ability both surfaces should be cleaned with a nonflammable household cleaning fluid.	When heated in water, this material loses its adherability. To restore, clean with nonflammable household solvent and bond before solvent evaporates.	See Kay Splint.
Working characteristics	This plastic has a large rubber content, giving it strong elastic memory. It softens over a wide temperature range, but it is at its most desirable at 160–170°F. The elastic memory makes it necessary for the therapist, while forming the splint, to hold it securely until the plastic is completely cool. The working time for this plastic when it is warm until it is completely cool is 8–10 min. This time can be accelerated by immersing the plastic in cold water. *Note:* San-Splint is translucent to x-rays (evident in an x-ray, but tissue is visible beneath the plastic).		See Kay Splint.

Kay Splint [2, 6]	Polyflex II [6]	Kay Splint-Isoprene [2, 6]	Aquaplast [7]
Beige	White	Beige	Powdery gold when cool
Rolyan Medical Products	Rolyan Medical Products	Rolyan Medical Products	WFR Aquaplast Corporation

(1) Splints with a great deal of curving contour, (2) splints that require a stretchy material, (3) splints with a large surface area, and (4) splints for burn patients. *Note:* The degree of rigidity in these materials mandates that care be exercised when making splints with a narrow area in a spot that receives stress. A splint made of narrow bars only should not be made from these materials.

Pen	Pen	Pen	Lead pencil
Scratch awl or nail	Scratch awl or nail	Scratch awl or nail	Scratch awl or nail

Because of low forming temperatures, it is impossible to sand or buff the edges of splints made from these plastics. The friction causes heat, which softens the plastic and the rubbing (as in sanding) will make the edges rougher instead of smoother. It is necessary, therefore, to cut the edges very smoothly with scissors or roll the edges down a very small distance to remove any roughness from the vicinity of the skin.

(1) *Be sure the working area is clean.* These materials have a relatively soft surface that picks up dirt. The dirt will detract from the aesthetic quality of the splint and make it difficult or impossible for the plastic to adhere to itself, as well as increase the chances for infection in an open wound. (2) Trace the pattern for the splint onto the plastic using the appropriate drawing device. (3) Heat the entire piece of plastic. (4) Cut out the splint carefully with scissors, using long smooth strokes, leaving the edges as smooth as possible. Care must be exercised to prevent the hot plastic from accidentally touching itself and adhering to itself in an undesirable spot. (5) Protect the patient's arm if necessary. (6) Reheat the cut out splint and form it. Make any necessary adjustments for fit. *Note:* The therapist must use hand lotion, Vaseline, or water on fingers when working with sticky surface Aquaplast, although WFR Aquaplast Corporation has made improvements in Aquaplast to reduce stickiness.

150–160°F (65–72°C)
These materials remain firm to 150°F, then become immediately moldable. The approximate heating time is 45 sec. If overheated there will be molding problems caused by excess stretching.

140°F (60°C)

Wet heat can be used effectively, and is often preferable, with these materials. A heat gun or other source of dry heat is often desirable to change small areas of the splint that must be adjusted. *Note:* The type of Aquaplast that has a sticky surface cannot be heated in an oven and must have an Aquaplast Frypan Guard in a skillet used with water to prevent the plastic from sticking to the skillet.

This material is coated on both surfaces to prevent sticking until it is wanted. Remember that the edges are not coated and are very adherent at all times. When it is desirable to have the surfaces stick, the surface of the cool material may be scraped with scissors, or both surfaces should be cleaned with a cleaning fluid containing methylene chloride. It is only necessary to heat one of the surfaces to be adhered, but if a very strong bond is wanted both surfaces may be heated.

The type of material with a coated surface is self-adherent (see Polyform).*

There is no rubber content in Polyform and Kay Splint, eliminating the elastic memory characteristic. When heated, Polyform and Kay Splint will drape with gravity, a characteristic that can be used as an advantage by forming splints with the arm held in the gravity-assisted position. Polyflex and Kay-Splint Isoprene have a small rubber content, giving them less drapability than Polyform and Kay Splint and more drapability than Orthoplast. There is some elastic memory in these materials, but not as much as Orthoplast. Because these materials do not soften until 150°F, accidental softening is unlikely. These materials cool rapidly, but harden slowly, making protection of the patient not as difficult while forming a splint on the patient's arm. The working time before hardening is 2–5 min. These materials can be autoclaved (sterilized) at a temperature below 140°F. They are translucent to x-rays (evident in x-ray, but one can see the tissue beneath the plastic). If undesirable marks from fingernails or something else occur in these materials, they can be rubbed smooth if the surface is heated.

Although there is some similarity to Polyform, Polyflex, and Orthoplast when using Aquaplast, it is necessary to study carefully the guidelines provided by the WFR Corporation. Among the 16 varieties of this product, working characteristics vary because of thickness, degree of elastic memory, tackiness of surface, and perforation.

*The type of Aquaplast with no coating has a sticky surface that adheres to everything, although this is supposed to have been reduced.

References

1. Cailliet, R. *Hand Pain and Impairment* (2nd ed.). Philadelphia: Davis, 1976.
2. Fred Sammons Inc. Catalog, P.O. Box 32, Brookfield, Illinois 60513
3. Johnson and Johnson Fact Sheet, Orthopedic Division, 501 George Street, New Brunswick, New Jersey 08903
4. Paramedical Distributors Fact Sheet, P.O. Box 19777, Kansas City, Missouri 64141
5. Rohm and Haas Company Fact Sheet, Independence Mall West, Philadelphia, Pennsylvania 19105
6. Rolyan Manufacturing Co., Inc. Fact Sheet, P.O. Box 555, 14635 Commerce Drive, Menomonee Falls, Wisconsin 53051
7. WFR Aquaplast Corporation Fact Sheet, 68 Birch Street, P.O. Box 215, Ramsey, New Jersey 07446

Suggested Reading

American Academy of Orthopaedic Surgeons. *Atlas of Orthotics.* St. Louis: Mosby, 1975.
Carl, T. K. B. Unpublished data, 1971. Revised by M. E. Fess and J. H. Kiel, 1973.
Malick, M. H. *Manual on Static Hand Splinting* (2nd ed.). Pittsburgh: Harmarville Rehabilitation Center, 1972.

COMMERCIAL SOURCES FOR SPLINTING SUPPLIES AND EQUIPMENT

Chattanooga Pharmacal Company
P.O. Box 4287
Chattanooga, Tennessee 37405

G.E. Miller, Inc.
484 South Broadway
Yonkers, New York 10705

Fred Sammons, Inc.
P.O. Box 32
Brookfield, Illinois 60513

Johnson and Johnson
Orthopedic Division
501 George Street
New Brunswick, New Jersey 08903

Paramedical Distributors
2020 Grand Avenue
P.O. Box 19777
Kansas City, Missouri 64141

J.A. Preston Corporation
71 Fifth Avenue
New York, New York 10003

Rohm and Haas
Independence Mall West
Philadelphia, Pennsylvania 19105

Rolyan Manufacturing Co., Inc.
P.O. Box 555
14635 Commerce Drive
Menomonee Falls, Wisconsin 53051

Smalley and Bates, Inc.
88 Park Avenue
Nutley, New Jersey 07110

Uniroyal Plastic Products
2638 N. Pulsaki Road
Chicago, Illinois 60639

WFR/Aquaplast Corporation
68 Birch Street
P.O. Box 215
Ramsey, New Jersey 07446

5. Construction and Forming Tips

Construction

It is very difficult to describe exactly how to construct a splint, as each person working on a splint has a slightly different technique to achieve the same or a similar result. The information in this chapter gives some very specific rules that must be followed to help ensure good results. Information is also offered to assist the beginner with where to start in making a splint and how to hold the plastic to form it. Some specific techniques that may help with completion of a splint are also explained.

1. *Curving contour* is important for maintaining strength in the splints. This contour is usually maintained because of the shape of the hand and forearm. There is no flat surface on the hand, which means that a well-fitting splint has no flat areas. With splints composed mostly of narrow bars or sections, care must be taken that a strong enough material is used and that as much curving contour as possible is included. With the increasing popularity of the less rigid plastics, many therapists are using tubes of the lower forming temperature plastic to increase the strength of narrow areas in splints.

   Some plastic materials have the ability to stretch when heated. These tend to be the ones with lower forming temperatures and to be softer and more pliable than the others, making the curving contour more essential. If contour is not molded into splints made from this type of material, the resulting splints will be somewhat flimsy. The stretchy quality makes it easier to obtain the desired curving contour in splints. It is also advisable with this type of material to be sure the splint has a large amount of surface area.

   The type of splint being made and how much curving contour is in the design of the splint in *all* areas play a large role in determining what type of plastic should be used.

2. With all types of plastic *smooth edges* are important for the patient's comfort, to prevent skin breakdown (even if the patient cannot feel it), for cosmesis, and to prevent stress, since even a small nick can lead to a crack.

   The methods for obtaining smooth edges vary with the specific materials being used. The more rigid plastics must have the edges finished with a file, sandpaper, and steel wool. The more flexible materials must be cut out with scissors, and this cut must be smooth. Some of the newer flexible materials can be heated slightly on the edges, and small rough areas can be rubbed away with the fingers. (See Chap. 4 for a discussion of which plastics have this quality.)

3. The proximal end of a volar, and sometimes a dorsal, splint should be slightly *lipped away from the skin* to prevent pressure (Fig. 5–1).

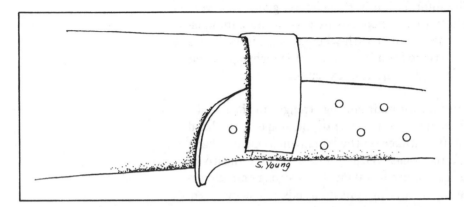

Figure 5-1. Lip the proximal end of the splint away from the arm.

4. When *bending* a material such as plastic, foam, or anything with some thickness, some of the size will be taken up with the bending. Usually it does not require a large excess in the pattern size, but some allowance must be made for this. This is important when making patterns and when cutting the splint out of plastic. The paper pattern must allow enough plastic material to curve around the hand and fit correctly. When making patterns it is usually not wise to add an extra amount around all the edges for the plastic to bend. However, if a therapist finds that it is difficult to get a splint to fit when the pattern fits well, then that therapist may need to make a habit of making patterns fit a little bit more loosely. When working with a plastic material that stretches, this characteristic is less significant, as with a splint that is too small a section of the plastic can sometimes be stretched to fit.

5. When using a rigid material (i.e., Kydex, Bioplastic, or Royalite) in an area that requires a sharp turn, it is sometimes necessary to notch the edge of the splint to allow the plastic to bend to the desired angle. When this is done the *notches must be U-shaped* rather than V-shaped to reduce the possibility of cracking the splint (Fig. 5–2). Remember, however, that this technique always reduces the strength of the splint, even when done correctly.

Figure 5-2. Notches should be U-shaped, as seen in the bottom splint. The V-shaped notches in the top splint will weaken the splint.

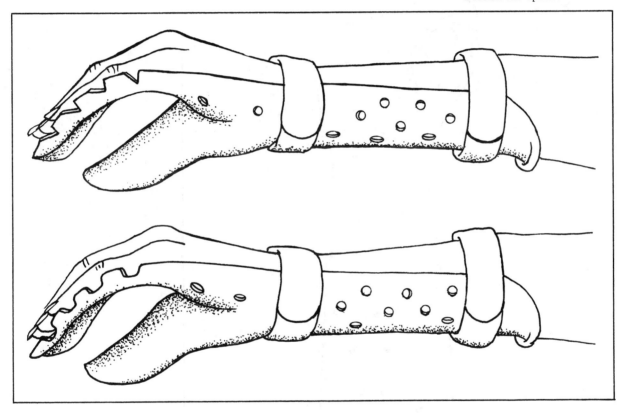

6. There are several instances when a *hole must be drilled in the plastic* to construct a splint. When this is necessary, the use of a low speed on the drill (if available) will help reduce friction that can heat the plastic and create many problems with rough spots and cosmesis. Any hole that is to be drilled needs to be center punched to prevent the drill bit from wandering and scratching the plastic.

7. When more than two *holes* must be drilled in a splint, they *should be staggered* to prevent a perforated edge type problem. This applies any time rivets or ventilation holes must be used in the splint (Fig. 5–3).

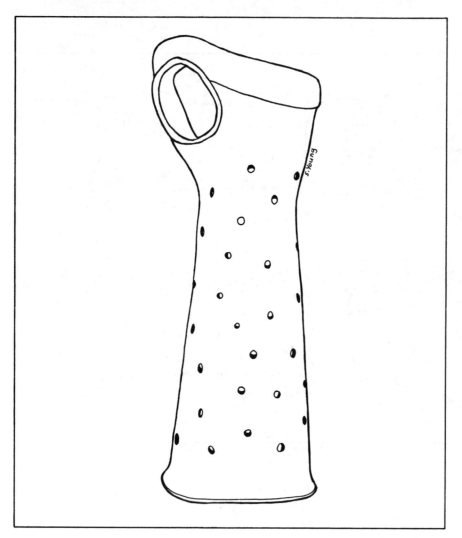

Figure 5-3. Correct placement of ventilation holes.

8. If two pieces of plastic must be riveted together, a *stable joint* will require two or more rivets. A *mobile joint* is made with just one rivet.

9. *When a cut terminates in the center of a rigid plastic,* a hole should be drilled at the end of the cut. An example of this can be seen in the resting pan splint at the thumb post. Placing a hole at the end of the cut makes smoothing the edges of the splint less troublesome and also disperses any stress placed on the splint around a circle rather than ending it abruptly in a point [1] (Fig. 5–4).

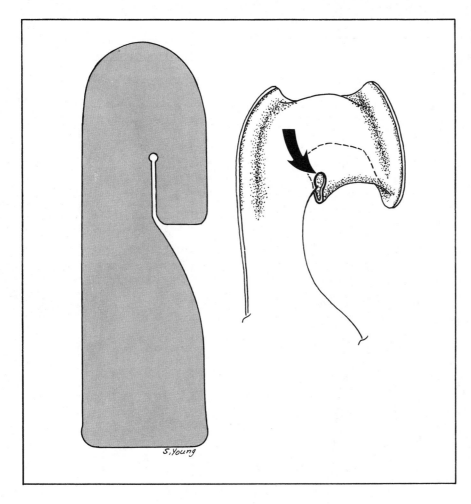

Figure 5-4. Drill a hole at the end of a cut that terminates in the middle of the plastic.

10. Any time a nonporous material, such as a plastic splint, is covering the skin, the patient is likely to have a perspiration problem. One of the techniques to help alleviate this problem is to put *ventilation holes* in the splint. An attempt to place these holes randomly should be made. If placed in a straight line, it is possible that they will weaken the splint in the same manner that a perforated edge makes paper more easily torn. They should be one inch from the edge of a splint and should be about 1½ inches from each other (see Fig. 5–3). Figure 5–5 shows ventilation holes that are much too numerous and too close together.

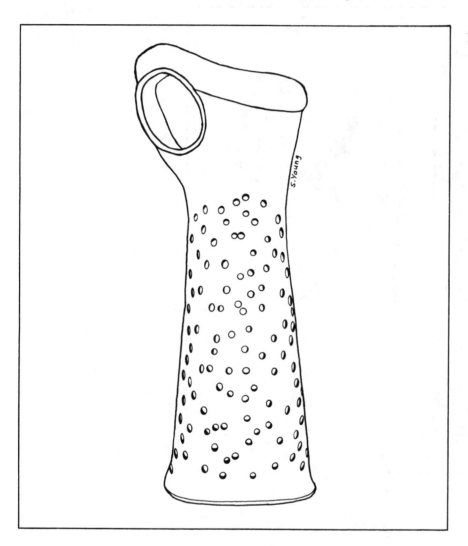

Figure 5-5. Incorrectly placed ventilation holes.

Plastic that can be purchased with ventilation holes already drilled is less desirable. The predrilled holes are usually placed in straight lines and too close together. Invariably holes end up on the edge of the splint, causing all the problems involved with the edges not being finished smoothly. In addition to these drawbacks, the preperforated plastic is more expensive than the plastic that can be ventilated as desired. Ventilation holes should be drilled *prior* to forming the splint when the splint is made of a *rigid nonstretchy material.* Ventilation holes should be drilled or punched with a leather punch *after* the splint is formed when stretchy material is used. This prevents the holes from becoming larger as the splint is formed.

11. *Padding a splint* should not be necessary. Padding to relieve pressure is ineffective since the pad will increase the pressure. Anything permanent added to line the splint will collect dirt and perspiration, increasing the possibility for skin breakdown. Any type of foam or plastic padding increases the heat that collects in the splint and negates any ventilation holes that are present.

    To combat the problem of heat, in addition to ventilation holes, a thin absorbent (sock type) lining may be used. This should be something that can be changed and washed regularly and not be a permanent part of the splint. A cotton "dress" glove, possibly with the fingers cut off, works well; a stockinette worn under the splint, or a cotton knee sock with the foot part cut off will also work. Another technique to combat the heat and perspiration is a spray deodorant or baby powder used on the hand. With small children, and a simply designed splint, sometimes a tissue inside the splint will do a great deal to increase the comfort of the splint and decrease the heat.

    If for some reason an exact lining is needed for the splint, the original pattern should be used. It is very difficult to cut a lining shaped correctly after the splint has been formed, unless the pattern is available.

12. It is important for the comfort of the patient, especially if any activity is to be accomplished while the splint is worn, that as much skin as the design of the splint will permit is left exposed for *sensation.*

13. If a splint is not *pleasing aesthetically* to a patient, it probably will not be worn.

14. If the patient has even a little bit of *function,* he will be very likely to prefer that to a splint that decreases function, even if it is the most well-made splint possible. A splint should show some visible improvement to the patient either immediately or very soon in order for it to be accepted.

15. Another factor that is important in determining whether the splint is worn has been termed *gadget tolerance* [2]. Some people can tolerate several external things in contact with their body while others will balk at even one piece of equipment. A therapist must acknowledge this and attempt to appease and work with a patient who has a low gadget tolerance.

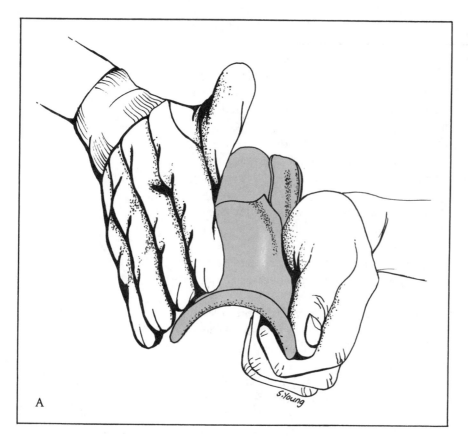

Figure 5-6A. Shaping a splint by stroking with the palm and fingers.

Forming a Splint

Forming a splint is a matter of heating the plastic to its forming temperature, moving it into the desired position, and cooling the splint in that position. Anyone who has ever made a splint understands that, although correct, this is very much an oversimplification. There are some steps to follow and precautions to take that will help in making the splint, as well as in improving its quality. This text does not give a step-by-step description of forming each splint, but rather a list of things that will help the splinter.

1. One of the most important facts to realize is that some forming can and should be done on the patient's hand, but some of the forming can and should be done with only the therapist's hands. This is accomplished by shaping with the whole hand, stroking with the palm and fingers, and using the table top (Figs. 5–6A, B).

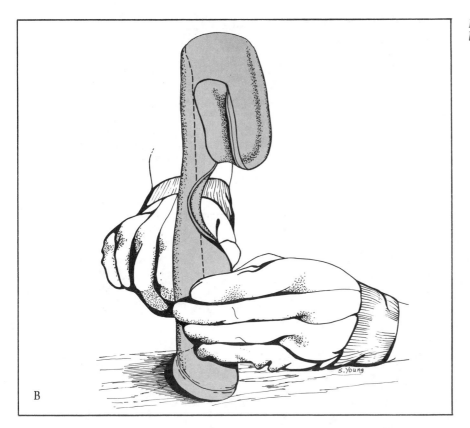

B

Figue 5-6B. Shaping a splint by using a table top.

2. When forming the splint, begin in the center and work toward the edges. This means that the first concern with almost every splint is the transverse arch support. After forming the arch support it is usually best to form the wrist extensor bar and the forearm bar, if the splint has these two parts. The third area to be formed should be the large parts in the hand area (i.e., finger pan, dorsal metacarpal bar, or deviation bars). The last things to be formed should be all of the small areas on the splint, which includes a **C** bar, a thumb post, an ulnar deviation bar, the longitudinal arch support, and any lipping that needs to be done to prevent pressure.

3. It is important to heat the plastic only in the area that needs to be moved. The reason that the smaller parts of the splint are formed last is because they heat quickly and can be easily lost while trying to get a larger area hot (see 2).

4. One procedure that will help in the effort to heat only the desired area, as well as speed up forming, is to be sure that the plastic is completely cool in one area before attempting to heat an adjacent area. If the hot plastic is not completely cooled prior to heating an adjacent section, the heat being applied will diffuse into the partially heated plastic, causing the shape that has been gained to be lost. A bucket of ice water in the working area will allow the therapist to plunge the splint or part of the splint into the water while supporting it in the correct position. Holding onto the hot plastic, or supporting it in some way, is an important part of this, as the ice and water can push the plastic out of shape on its way into the water. If the tap water in the area is very cold, it can be used with the same precaution; the running water can change the shape of unsupported hot plastic.

5. When using the heat gun, learn how to aim the heat so that only the part of the plastic that needs to move is being heated.

a. One way to do this is to keep the part of the splint that is to remain cool behind the nozzle (Fig. 5–7A).

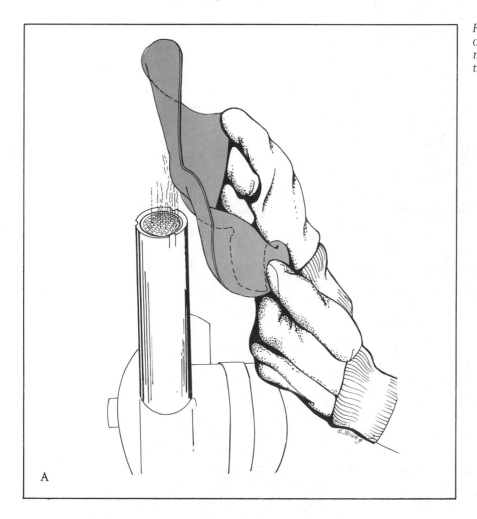

Figure 5-7A. Hold the portion of the splint that is not being moved behind the nozzle of the heat gun.

A

b. Another technique is to cover the part of the splint that is to remain cool with the therapist's hand. If the therapist then keeps from burning his or her hand, the splint section will stay cool.

c. Remember that curved plastic acts as a trough, which directs any heat through it into undesirable areas unless care is used to direct it to an area that is not vulnerable (Fig. 5–7B).

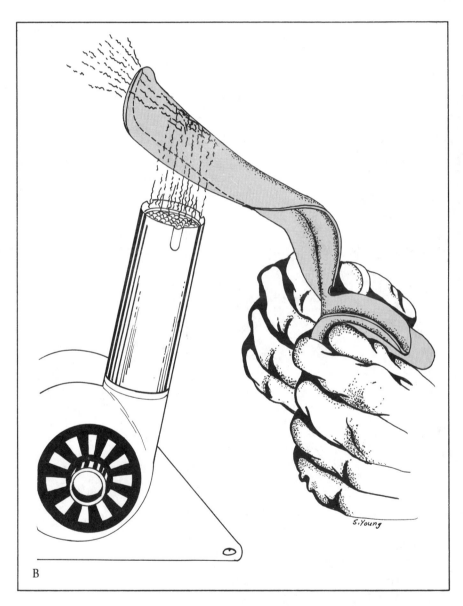

B

Figure 5-7B. Remember that curved portions of the splint act as a trough that can direct the heat to undesirable areas. This illustration shows the heat being directed away from the center of the splint so that it will not create problems.

   d. Hold the part to be heated about one inch from the nozzle. If it is held further from the nozzle, the heat becomes less intense as it cools in the room air and it diffuses into a wider space. Holding the plastic about one inch from the nozzle causes the desired part of the plastic to heat more rapidly and prevents heat from reaching undesirable areas (Fig. 5–7C).

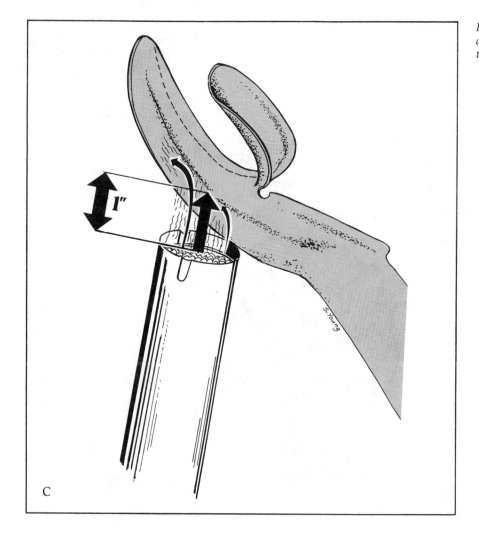

Figure 5-7C. Hold the splint about one inch from the nozzle of the heat gun.

   6. Turn the splint over while heating it to direct heat onto both sides of the plastic. If the therapist attempts to thoroughly heat the entire thickness of plastic without turning it, the possibility of burning the plastic before it becomes moldable becomes almost a certainty.

   7. When attempting to move a section of a splint, the entire section, plus ¼–½ inch all around the section, needs to be heated. This allows the shaping to blend into the rest of the splint and avoids sharp angles, which is something that no hand has.

   8. Remember to include the transverse metacarpal arch in all hand splints, but make it fit the individual client. A very large, deep arch may look attractive, but if the client has a shallow arch, it will cause pressure. If the transverse metacarpal arch is causing pressure there are several things that can be checked in addition to whether the client has a shallow or a deep arch.

a. One of these things is to note whether the splint is to be worn during activity or rest. A hand at rest has a more shallow arch than one in use. A splint to be worn during sleep can be quite uncomfortable if it has an extremely deep transverse metacarpal arch. Unless there is a specific reason that the physician has required a client to have a deep arch in his splint, a flatter arch is better for a splint to be worn during rest.

b. Notice that the transverse metacarpal arch does not just go up into the hand. When the hand is held in pronation in a functional position, it curves both up and down from a flat plane that is drawn through it. The center of the palm is above the plane as one would expect with the transverse metacarpal arch, but both the radial and ulnar sides are below the flat plane. Sometimes it is necessary to push the radial and ulnar side of the transverse metacarpal arch down in order to have it give the necessary fit and eliminate pressure (Fig. 5–8).

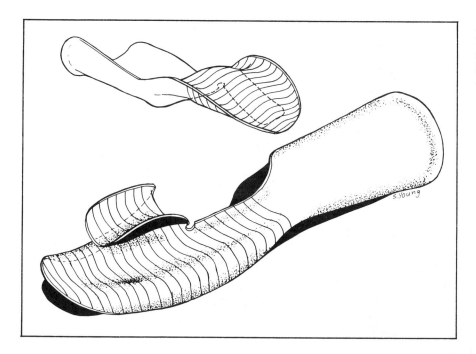

Figure 5-8. The curve of the transverse metacarpal arch goes up and down from a flat plane drawn through the hand.

9. If the wrist is to be placed in a neutral position rather than in extension with a volar splint, the transverse metacarpal arch support is still present and should push the palm dorsally. However, proximal to the transverse metacarpal arch area and distal to the axis of the wrist joint (the lay term for this area is the heel of the hand) there is a small area of muscle, tendon, carpal bone, and other tissue that must be allowed for in the splint by pushing the plastic down volarly (Fig. 5–9). When doing this the therapist may think that the wrist is flexing, but if a goniometer is used, it can be seen that the wrist is actually in neutral. If for some reason a splint must be positioned in flexion, the bulk of the heel of the hand is again important in the same way.

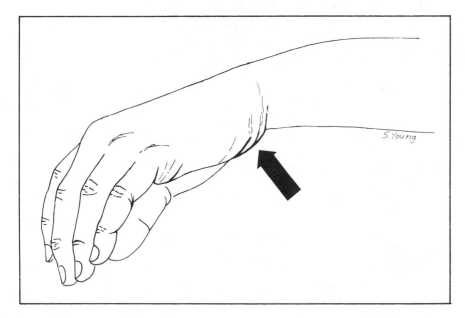

Figure 5-9. If the wrist is positioned in neutral or flexion, the heel of the hand often must receive special attention to avoid pressure on it.

10. There is a temptation, when using the plastics that adhere to themselves, to roll up and stick down any area that is too long, too wide, or not quite right. This can lead to sections of the splint having several layers (sometimes as many as four or more) stuck together. This practice should be avoided. If this is done, and for some reason the splint needs to be reshaped in that area, then in order to get the plastic hot clear though, it must be heated much higher than the forming temperature on the outside layers, making the chances of burning the patient, therapist, or plastic itself very high.

11. When finishing a splint, avoid leaving tiny holes or narrow places that cannot be washed thoroughly. People who wear splints are likely to get their hands dirty and sweaty in the same way that people who do not wear splints get their hands dirty. In addition to that, they will often be somewhat uncoordinated, if for no other reason than that they are wearing a splint. A splint that cannot be washed well becomes intolerable owing to the dirt, sweat, and food that is trapped in small holes. This dirt can cause multiple problems such as pressure sores, infection, or the splint not being worn.

References
1. American Academy of Orthopaedic Surgeons. *Atlas of Orthotics.* St. Louis: Mosby, 1975.
2. Anderson, M. H. *Upper Extremity Orthotics.* Springfield, Ill.: Thomas, 1965.

Suggested Reading
American Academy of Orthopaedic Surgeons. *Atlas of Orthotics.* St. Louis: Mosby, 1975.
Anderson, M. H. *Upper Extremity Orthotics.* Springfield, Ill.: Thomas, 1965.
Carl, T. K. B. Unpublished data, 1971. Revised by M. E. Fess and J. H. Kiel, 1973.
Institute and Workshop on Hand Splinting Construction. Pittsburgh: Harmarville Rehabilitation Center, March 9–11, June 2, 1967.
Malick, M. H. *Manual on Dynamic Hand Splinting with Thermoplastic Materials.* Pittsburgh: Harmarville Rehabilitation Center, 1974.

6. Straps and Closures

Many different materials can be used effectively for splint straps. These include such things as webbing, leather, elastic, cloth, Ace bandages, dressings, and Velcro tape. The width of the strap depends on where it is used on the splint and the size of the person being splinted. Note that a wider strap distributes the pressure over a wide area and gives a better purchase to position the limb.

Except when using Velcro tape for the strap, a separate type of closure must be used to hold the strap together. In addition to Velcro tape, other types of closures available are tape, buckles, safety pins, and studs.

Although it is occasionally more expensive (therapist time in fabrication must be included when figuring this cost), Velcro tape is by far the easiest thing to use for straps and closures. There are also completed straps available (Velstrap is the one sold by Smalley and Bates, Inc., distributors of Velcro brand products) that have the strap and closure bonded together so that the therapist can simply attach it to the splint with no extra work. These completed straps, of course, add even more to the cost of the strap.

When used as a closure, the Velcro fastener consists of two tapes. One of the tapes is a series of small hooks; this tape is called hook tape. The other tape is a mass of small loops; this tape is called napped loop tape. When pressed together, the hooks become embedded in the loops, creating a strong bond that can be easily peeled apart [3] (Fig. 6–1). The load on the Velcro closure can be reduced by one-half by using a rope and pulley system. In order to do this the strap is passed through a D-ring and laid back on itself, with the loose end attached to the original portion by mating the Velcro portions [1] (Fig. 6–2).

When employing Velcro as a strap, the part that wraps around the arm should usually be the napped loop tape, which is generally soft enough that no additional protection is needed next to the patient's skin. Velcro hook tape is then stuck to the surface of the splint, keeping it from contacting the patient and causing discomfort. If it is not desirable to use Velcro napped loop tape for the strap, webbing, elastic, or cloth may be used for the strap with napped loop tape sewn on each end for the closure.

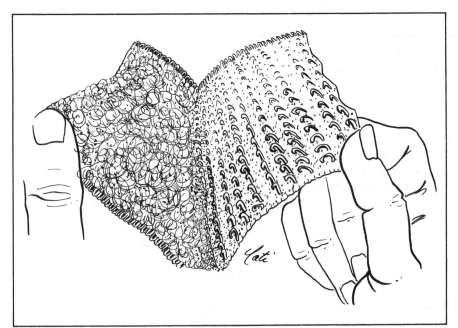

Figure 6-1. Velcro consists of one tape with many small hooks that become embedded in the numerous loops that are on a second tape.

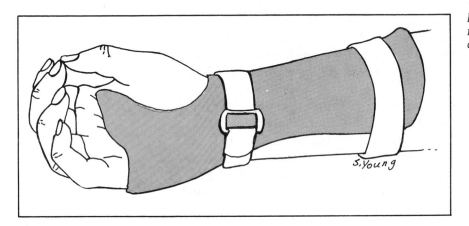

Figure 6-2. The use of a D-ring reduces the load on a Velcro closure by one-half.

Application of Velcro to a Splint
Standard Backing
Both hook tape and napped loop tape can be purchased with nylon material as the only backing. In order to stick this type of Velcro to a splint one of the types of Velcro liquid adhesive must be used. The Velcro napped loop tape is most often used with standard backing since usually it is not necessary to stick it to anything. Standard backing is also the type required when the Velcro is to be sewn to anything.

Adhesive Backed Velcro
Adhesive backing is offered on either the hook tape or the napped loop tape. Solvent activated backed tapes are one type of adhesive backing that is available. The most useful adhesive backing for splinting, however, is *Pressure Sensitive Adhesive Backing.* This backing has a tacky surface on the back side, with release paper protecting it until it is ready for use. When using it, the release paper is removed and the Velcro tape is placed where desired. This type of adhesive backing works well *one time.* It is important that the release paper is not removed until just before placing it on the splint, that it is placed where it is wanted, and that it will not need to be removed. It is often convenient to purchase Velcro hook tape with pressure sensitive adhesive backing, as this is the type of tape that is usually stuck to a splint.

When sticking the Velcro hook tape to the splint, it is best to use a single strip across the width of the splint so that the napped loop tape strap hooks to both sides of the hook tape and pulls the closure onto the splint more tightly. If two tabs are used on either side of the splint for a closure, it may be necessary to rivet them in place since any stress placed on the strap puts pressure on the tabs to come off (Fig. 6–3).

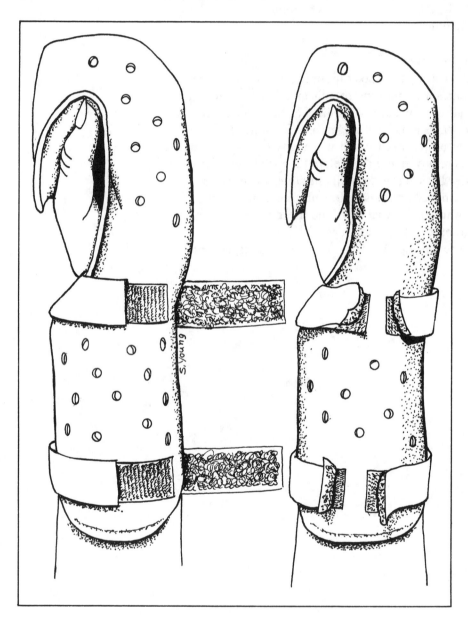

Figure 6-3. It is better to use a single strip of hook tape (left) than to use two tabs of hook tape (right).

Be sure that the Velcro is put on flat with no air bubbles under it and that the Velcro tape does not extend past the edge of the splint (Fig. 6-4). This will ensure that the Velcro hook tape stays in place.

Patients appreciate all of the Velcro hook closure being covered with Velcro napped loop tape strap when the splint is in place. Any hook tape that is left exposed will collect dirt and will catch in hosiery, sweaters, and knit clothing. This also helps the patient know how tight to fasten the splint on his arm, as he needs only to make the two ends of the strap meet each other.

To prevent the strap from being lost, it may be desirable to put a spot of Velcro liquid adhesive between the closure of Velcro hook tape and Velcro napped loop tape on one side of the splint. When hardened, this prevents that side from opening. Usually it is best to glue the closure on the ulnar side of the splint so that the patient is able to apply and remove the splint without help. (The radial side of the patient's arm is more accessible than the ulnar side, especially if the strap must be applied and removed with the teeth.) If the patient has bilateral splints, special steps may need to be taken (such as loops on the end of the strap) for the patient to be able to apply and remove the splints independently.

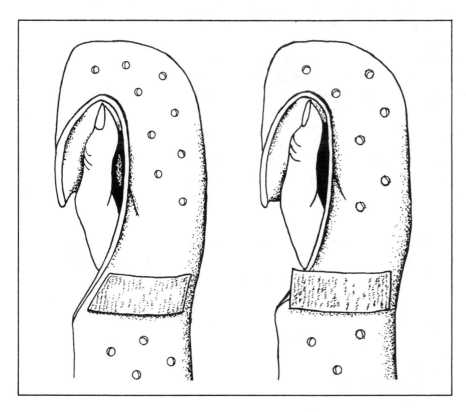

Figure 6-4. The Velcro hook tape should not extend past the edge of the splint. The splint on the left shows the Velcro hook tape placed correctly.

When working with children (or a dependent adult), it is sometimes necessary to reverse procedures and make self-application and self-removal more difficult.

Other Strapping Materials

Materials other than Velcro that may be used for straps include the following.

Webbing is a popular, inexpensive strapping material. It may be purchased in various widths and cut to the desired length. The closures that may be used are Velcro sewn to the ends, a buckle, or a safety pin. If the webbing is very sturdy, it may be possible to close it with a stud.

Leather has been used for straps for many years and is the strongest strapping material. The best closures to use with a leather strap are buckles or studs. It is difficult, though possible, to use Velcro as a closure.

Elastic is frequently used with an orthokinetic splint. The elastic is used in various widths to suit the purpose of the splint. The continual stretching and contracting of the elastic over the muscle bellies serves as a facilitator to strengthen the muscle over which it lies. Velcro is usually the best closure to use with elastic, because often a three-inch, or more, width of elastic must be used to fulfill the purpose of the splint, and Velcro can be adapted more easily to greater widths [2].

Cloth may be sewn to any width and length desired to provide a large strap. It is usually best to use material that does not stretch to be sure that the splint is held in exactly the correct position, and to avoid any undesirable facilitation as described with elastic. Again because of the width, Velcro is usually the best closure to use with cloth straps.

Ace bandages or dressings may be used to hold a splint in place. Because of the heat and lack of cosmesis, these should be used only if the patient must wear the ace bandage or dressing for some other reason. The closure for these two materials may be tape, a safety pin, or a hook arrangement provided with the Ace bandage (Fig. 6–5).

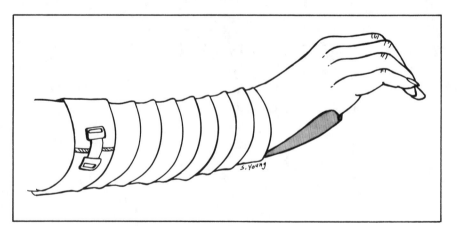

Figure 6-5. Sometimes an Ace bandage is used to hold a splint in place.

Closures

Many people are familiar with the closures that have been mentioned, with the possible exception of Velcro. Illustrations of closures not shown earlier are provided here in lieu of a written description of them (Figs. 6–6, 6–7, 6–8).

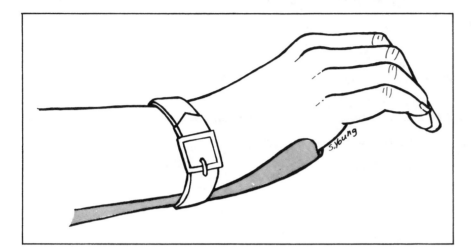

Figure 6-6. Buckle closure.

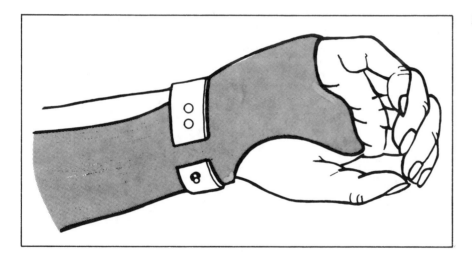

Figure 6-7. Stud closure.

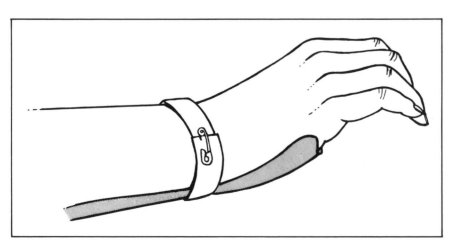

Figure 6-8. Safety pin closure.

References

1. American Academy of Orthopaedic Surgeons. *Atlas of Orthotics.* St. Louis: Mosby, 1975.
2. Farber, S. D. *Neurorehabilitation: A Multisensory Approach.* Philadelphia: Saunders, 1982.
3. Smalley and Bates, Inc. Velcro Brand Fastening Systems, 88 Park Avenue, Nutley, New Jersey 07110. Technical data sheets.

Suggested Reading

American Academy of Orthopaedic Surgeons. *Atlas of Orthotics.* St. Louis: Mosby, 1975.

Carl, T. K. B. Unpublished data, 1971. Revised by M. E. Fess and J. H. Kiel, 1973.

Farber, S. D. *Neurorehabilitation: A Multisensory Approach.* Philadelphia: Saunders, 1982.

Fred Sammons, Inc. *Be OK! Professional Self-Help Aids Catalog.* Box 32, Brookfield, Ill. 60513, 1980.

Smalley and Bates, Inc. Velcro Brand Fastening Systems, 88 Park Avenue, Nutley, New Jersey 07110. Technical data sheets.

Activities to ensure efficient and effective splinting include evaluating the splint, pricing the splint, and writing a note about the splint in the patient's medical record.

Evaluating the Splint

The process of splinting involves continual and repeated evaluation. As the splint is formed the therapist must look at each part to see that it is correct in every aspect, as well as how each part might affect every other part's correctness.

A therapist is often asked to examine a splint extemporaneously and must know immediately what to look for in examination.

Using the list of questions below, static splints can be evaluated comprehensively. It may be noted that there is some repetition when using this list, as the splint parts often have more than one function; also, each part affects the whole.

1. Is the splint necessary for this patient?
2. Does the splint effectively fulfill its purpose?
3. Has an appropriate material been used for the splint?
4. Is the workmanship of good quality? Cosmesis? Burn spots? Smooth edges? Sufficient curving contour for strength?
5. Does the splint hold the joints it supports in a functional position, or in a position that is appropriate for the patient's diagnosis?
6. Is dual obliquity evident in the splint, and does it fit the dual obliquity of the patient's hand?
7. Does the splint support the arches that it covers in the hand?
8. Does the patient experience any pain either initially or after wearing and using the splint for several minutes?
9. Are there any areas of the splint that look as though they might cause pressure (whether or not they cause pain) as the patient wears or uses the splint?
10. As the patient wears and uses the splint does it remain in the proper position without frequent manual adjustments by the patient or another person?
11. Are all the axes of joints in the splint positioned correctly at the axes of the joints in the hand?
12. Is the desired motion available or eliminated at the wrist, MP, PIP, and DIP joints of the hand?
13. Do the prehension patterns that remain with the splint in place work effectively for the patient?
14. Are all of the parts of the splint positioned correctly for the best fit, leverage, comfort, and to fulfil their purpose?
15. Do all the splint parts maintain all the hand parts in the correct position?
16. Are all the parts used in the splint necessary for this particular patient?
17. Is the patient aware of the purpose of the splint, how to use the splint, and how to care for the splint?
18. Can the patient (or other responsible person) correctly apply and remove the splint? How quickly?

Pricing Splints

In order to determine cost, one must consider the expense of the materials. This is done by figuring exactly how much of each type material was used and then totaling these expenses. A patient should be charged for any scraps of material created in the making of his splint that could not possibly be used to make something else. The plastic can be figured as cost per square inch. Most other materials can be figured at cost per inch or cost per single item.

After figuring the cost of the materials, the time used by the therapist is added. Often this is the same rate used for any other treatment given in the clinic. (Usually this rate will include depreciation of permanent equipment in the department used in the fabrication of splints.) The charge is frequently based on the time required by an experienced therapist to complete the splint. If excess time caused by the patient or diagnosis is used, it should be included in the charge. The inexperience of a therapist in making splints should not jeopardize the patient cost.

A price for splints that are made frequently can be prepared in advance by averaging the cost of materials and time used in construction, thus avoiding a detailed calculation on each splint made. This allows the clinic to have a standard price list for common splints (Fig. 7–1).

Splint Note Writing in the Medical Record

When writing a note in a patient's medical record about a splint, the same rules that apply to all professional writing should be used. In regard to the splint itself, the following list of facts must be included.

1. Patient's name: The *complete* name should be included on every separate piece of paper used in the note, either as a stamped heading or in the body of the note, or both.
2. Patient's age.
3. Patient's sex, race, and ambulatory status: These items may not always be applicable and can be eliminated, but should be included if they in any way affect the treatment or diagnosis of the patient.
4. Diagnosis.
5. Date and reason for referral to occupational therapy.
6. Patient's position prior to splinting, including range of motion and muscle tone.
7. Patient's position after splinting instead of, or in addition to, the name of the splint.
8. Date the splint was delivered to the patient.
9. Type of plastic, straps, closures, and other materials used in the splint.
10. Description (use a drawing if necessary) of anything unusual about the splint, either in design or construction.
11. How the splint is to be worn or not worn.
12. When the splint is to be worn or not worn.
13. Exercises or other activities to augment the wear of the splint.
14. The fact that the purpose, care and use of the splint was explained to the patient, family, hospital staff and/or other appropriate people; and the fact that these people understood the process and demonstrated the ability to carry it out.
15. How well the patient tolerated the splint.

Figure 7-1. To determine the cost of the resting pan splint shown here, the therapist must total the cost of the plastic, the straps, and the construction time.

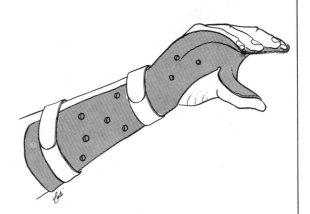

Plastic

Sold in sheets: 18 × 24 in.
Cost of one sheet: $25.00
Section of plastic used: 7 × 18 in.

$$
\begin{array}{r}
18 \text{ in.} \\
\times 24 \text{ in.} \\
\hline
432 \text{ Sq. in. per sheet}
\end{array}
\qquad
\begin{array}{r}
18 \text{ in.} \\
\times 7 \text{ in.} \\
\hline
126 \text{ Sq. in. of plastic used}
\end{array}
$$

$$
\begin{array}{r}
\$\ .058 \text{ Cost per sq. in.} \\
432 \overline{)\$25.00}
\end{array}
$$

$$
\begin{array}{r}
126 \text{ Sq. in.} \\
\times .058 \text{ Cost per sq. in.} \\
\hline
\$7.30 = \text{Cost of plastic used}
\end{array}
$$

Straps

1-in. Velcro straps used throughout
10 yd. standard backed, napped loop tape cost: $11.00
Napped loop tape used: 18 in.
10 yd. pressure sensitive adhesive backed, hook tape cost: $18.50
Hook tape used: 8 in.
360 in. = 10 yd.

$$
\begin{array}{r}
\$\ .031 \text{ Cost per in. of napped loop tape} \\
360 \overline{)\$11.00}
\end{array}
$$

$$
\begin{array}{r}
\$.031 \\
\times 18 \text{ in.} \\
\hline
\$.558 \text{ Cost of napped loop tape used}
\end{array}
$$

$$
\begin{array}{r}
\$\ .051 \text{ Cost per in. of hook tape} \\
360 \overline{)\$18.50}
\end{array}
$$

$$
\begin{array}{r}
\$.051 \\
\times 8 \text{ in.} \\
\hline
\$.408 \text{ Cost of hoop tape used}
\end{array}
$$

$$
\begin{array}{r}
\$.558 \text{ Napped loop tape} \\
+.408 \text{ Hook tape} \\
\hline
\$.966 \text{ or } \$.97 = \text{Total cost of Velcro used}
\end{array}
$$

Construction time

Average time necessary: 45 min.
Fifteen minute treatment charge: $12.00

$$
\begin{array}{r}
\$12.00 \\
\times\ 3 \\
\hline
\$36.00 \text{ Cost of therapist time}
\end{array}
$$

Cost of resting pan splint

$$
\begin{array}{r}
\$\ 7.30 \text{ Plastic} \\
.97 \text{ Straps} \\
36.00 \text{ Construction time} \\
\hline
\$44.27 \text{ Cost of splint}
\end{array}
$$

Round off to $45.00.

Occasionally there is a valid reason for omitting one or more of these items. If this is done, the item should still be mentioned (except as noted in 3) with the reason for omission (e.g., "Complete range of motion and muscle tone was not completed on the initial visit because the physician requested that this be delayed until after the splint was completed and worn for twenty-four hours.").

In a clinic where a large number of splints are constructed on a regular basis, it will be necessary to simplify and shorten the note writing process. One way to maintain accurate, responsible records and not spend many hours writing notes is to use standardized forms.

Items 1 through 4 (except ambulatory status) can be furnished with a stamping card that may already be used by the facility housing the occupational therapy clinic. Items 6 and 7 can be handled with a standard evaluation form that can be filled out during the evaluation itself while the patient is present. Parts of items 9 and 10 can be handled by descriptive forms of the common splints made in the clinic. Either one of the forms can be included in the patient chart, or a statement can be made that a certain type of splint was made and a more complete description may be obtained by contacting the occupational therapy department. Item 13 can be handled with one list of exercises and how they are to be executed, with the specific ones to be used by the individual patient marked accordingly or several different exercise pages with only the appropriate ones given to a particular patient. Items 11, 12, and 14 can be handled with care and usage forms prepared in advance for specific splints. The appropriate forms can be used for a specific patient.

If forms are made for exercises and care and use of a splint, they can be used to instruct the patient and provide a written explanation, as well as simplify the writing of notes. By using all five of the above techniques, the therapist is left addressing only items 5, 8, and 15.

The following are samples of some forms (Figs. 7-2 through 7-6) that are used. These forms were contributed by the pediatric Occupational Therapy Department at James Whitcomb Riley Hospital for Children, Indiana University Medical Center, Indianapolis, Indiana and by the Occupational Therapy Department at Saint Francis Hospital Center, Beech Grove, Indiana.

General Splint Care Form

1. Purpose of splint:
2. Application of splint:
3. Wearing time:
4. Wash splint in cold water using mild detergent. Do not place splint near any source of heat (e.g., direct sunlight, radiator).
5. Observe carefully for skin irritation or redness that lasts more than 30 minutes after splint removal. If these problems occur, contact your therapist immediately.
6. Baby powder or stockinette worn under the splint may help prevent perspiration problems.
7. Have splint reevaluated by therapist at _____
   If questions or problems arise regarding splints, please contact me.

Therapist:
Occupational Therapy Department
Riley Hospital for Children
1100 West Michigan Street, Room A402
Indianapolis, IN 46223
(317) 264-8211

Figure 7-2. General splint care form, Riley Hospital for Children.

Care of a Resting Pan Splint

_____ has been provided with a splint to hold the wrist up and the fingers out straight. If this splint is worn according to the doctor's instructions, tightening that could immobilize the hand may be prevented.
   Every day the splint should be cleaned with *cold* water and soap.
How to put the splint on:
1. Be sure the splint is clean.
2. When putting on, be sure the wrist strap is exactly over the wrist, and the thumb platform has its curve as far back as possible in the space between the first finger and thumb.
3. Fasten the wrist strap first.
4. Then fasten the other straps.
5. It will be more comfortable for your child if he or she wears the top of a sock, stockinette, or a very thin piece of gauze.
6. If there is any problem with perspiration, baby powder or a dry spray deodorant (e.g., Calm) may be used.

   If there is any problem with the splint at any time please call me at (317) 264-8211, or write to:

Therapist:
Riley Hospital for Children
Occupational Therapy Department
1100 West Michigan Street, Room A402
Indianapolis, IN 46223
(317) 264-8211

Specific instructions:

Figure 7-3. Care of a resting pan splint, Riley Hospital for Children.

St. Francis Hospital Center
Occupational Therapy Department
783-8111 or 783-8113

Hand Rehabilitation Program

Patient's name: _____ Date: _____

Each circled exercise is specifically indicated for your hand problem. Following your hand program as outlined will be to your benefit.

Hand program:
A: _____
B: _____

Exercises: (active/passive range-of-motion exercises)
1. Wrist:
    1. Bend the wrist forward, back, and side to side with the unaffected hand.
    2. Grasp the _____ wrist with the _____ hand. Straighten both arms, assisting with the unaffected arm.
    3. Push away from the wall with your hands.
    4. With hand sideways, slide ____ lb. weight back and forth ____ times.
    5. With palms flat on tabletop, bend wrist back ____ times.
    6. With palms flat on tabletop, raise the forearm, bending the wrist back.
    7. With the wrist over edge of table and palm up, lift ____ lb. weight ____ times.
    8. With wrist over edge of table and palm down, lift ____ lb. weight ____ times.
    9. Close fingers into a tight fist and open.
    10. Turn a door handle. (May be given resistance by someone holding the other side of the handle.)
    11. Turn screws.

2. Forearm:
    1. With elbow tucked into your side and bent about 90 degrees, turn forearm, bringing palm up and then down.

(**Note:** Perform each exercise ____ times unless otherwise indicated.)

Figure 7-4. Exercise program form, St. Francis Hospital Center.

St. Francis Hospital Center
1600 Albany Street
Beech Grove, Indiana 46107
Occupational Therapy Department
783-8113 or 783-8111

Hand Rehabilitation Program

Patient's Name: _____ Date: _____

Do each exercise ten (10) times

Hand exercises:
1. Bend and straighten all fingers of the affected hand. Assist with the un-affected hand.
2. Touch each fingertip with the thumb, making an "O". Keep the other three fingers as straight as possible.
3. With palm flat on table, spread fingers apart and back together.
4. Blocking exercise: secure thumb at base of joint with the index finger on top of joint; bend the joint.
5. With palm flat on table, cup the hand.
6. With palm flat on table, raise and lower each finger.
7. With palm flat on table, touch the top of the adjacent finger.
8. With palm up, touch the table top with fingernails.
9. Touch the base of your palm with the fingertips.
10. With hand positioned on its side, position the thumb in front of the index finger and move the thumb in and out parallel with the table.
11. Isolate joints with the bunnell block and bend fingers.
12. Pick up coins or buttons of assorted sizes.
13. Place the pencil or putty in the palm and roll along the palm with the fingers.
14. Flip beads off fingertips.
15. Straighten thumb out like a hitchhiker, then bend across the palm.
16. Exercise with the traction glove.
17. Sand a dowel rod.
18. Activities: play checkers or chess, pick-up sticks, cut with scissors, tie knots, type, play piano, sew, shuffle and turn cards, and sand.
19. Carry book between thumb and fingers.
20. With washcloth on table top, use fingertips to draw the cloth together.
21. Interlace fingers, turn palms out.
22. With palms together, spread fingers apart and together, assisting with the unaffected hand.
23. Squeeze the foam piece.

Figure 7-5. Hand exercises form, St. Francis Hospital Center.

Figure 7-6. Patient instruction form, St. Francis Hospital Center.

St. Francis Hospital Center
Occupational Therapy Department

Hand Rehabilitation Program

Patient's Name: _____ Date: _____

Hand therapy schedule:
_____ Keep the arm elevated _____
_____ Massage with cocoa butter
_____ Perform the forearm/wrist exercises
_____ Perform the hand exercises   _____ minute sessions
_____ Perform the putty exercises _____
_____ Wear your _____ splint _____ times a day for _____ minute sessions
_____ Wear your _____ splint _____ times a day for _____ minute sessions
_____ Wear your _____ through the night
_____ Perform your desensitization techniques
_____ Additional comments: _____
_____
_____

Precautions (please watch for these possible problem areas):

1. Increased swelling: Elevate the arm, and massage
2. Decreased circulation: Massage, reposition
3. Increased joint pain following exercise: Do not exercise for _____
4. Your splint breaks: Make an appointment for splint adjustment
5. The splint results in increased pain: Do not wear the splint at your next appointment

If you should have any questions or problems, please feel free to contact your occupational therapist at the hospital between the hours of 8:00 A.M. and 4:30 P.M.

_____   Telephone number: 783-8113 or 783-8111
            Occupational therapist

Please bring these sheets to each appointment.

Suggested Reading

Carl, T. K. B. Unpublished data, 1971. Revised by M. E. Fess and J. H. Kiel, 1973.

O'Connor, J. R. Medical Aspects of Splinting. In E. R. Mayerson (Ed.), *Splinting Theory and Fabrication*. Clarence Center, N.Y.: Goodrich Printing and Lithographers, 1971.

For those individuals who wish to attain a more in-depth knowledge of the hand and its rehabilitation the following reading is suggested.

Historical Perspective

As in all subjects, splinting has its classic literature. All of these books are excellent and highly recommended for foundation reading.

American Academy of Orthopaedic Surgeons. *Orthopaedic Appliances Atlas, Volume 1.* Ann Arbor, Mich.: J.W. Edwards, 1952.

American Academy of Orthopaedic Surgeons. *Atlas of Orthotics.* St. Louis: C.V. Mosby, 1975.

Anderson, M. H. *Upper Extremity Orthotics.* Springfield, Ill.: Charles C. Thomas, 1965.

Boyes, J. H. *Bunnell's Surgery of the Hand.* Philadelphia: J.B. Lippincott, 1970.

Capener, N. The hand in surgery. *J. Bone Joint Surg.* 38B(1):128, 1956.

Licht, S. *Orthotics Etcetera.* Baltimore: Waverly, 1966.

Nickel, V. L., Perry, J., and Snelson, R. *Handbook of Handsplints.* Downey, Calif.: Rancho Los Amigos Hospital.

Hand Anatomy

If a therapist is to be effective working on a hand rehabilitation team, a thorough knowledge of the anatomy of the hand is essential. The following books can all help in this area.

Johnson, M. K. *The Hand Book.* Springfield, Ill.: Charles C. Thomas, 1973.

Johnson, M. K., and Cohen, M. J. *The Hand Atlas.* Springfield, Ill.: Charles C. Thomas, 1975.

Rasch, P. J., and Burke, R. K. *Kinesiology and Applied Anatomy* (6th ed.). Philadelphia: Lea and Febiger, 1978.

Hand Rehabilitation

The following books were written by surgeons and intended to be read by surgeons. For a therapist to learn the physician's point of view in regard to specific hand problems is a tremendous advantage. In addition, the books by Caillet and Wynn Parry both have sections discussing the importance of splints and therapists in the treatment of hand problems.

Byrne, J. J. *The Hand: Its Anatomy and Diseases.* Springfield, Ill.: Charles C. Thomas, 1959.

Cailliet, R. *Hand Pain and Impairment* (2nd ed.). Philadelphia: F.A. Davis Company, 1976.

Wynn Parry, C. B. *Rehabilitation of the Hand* (3rd ed.). London: Butterworth, 1973.

Splinting

Various viewpoints and philosophies of splinting, in addition to discussions of some specific treatments for specific problems, are offered in the following books.

Barr, N. *The Hand: Principles and Techniques of Simple Splint Making in Rehabilitation.* Boston: Butterworth, 1975.

Fess, E. E., Gettle, K. S., and Strickland, J. W. *Hand Splinting Principles and Methods.* St. Louis: C.V. Mosby, 1981.

Hollis, L. I. Hand Rehabilitation. In H. L. Hopkins and H. D. Smith (Eds.), *Willard and Spackman's Occupational Therapy* (5th ed.). Philadelphia: J.B. Lippincott, 1978.

Malick, M. H. *Manual on Static Hand Splinting* (2nd ed.). Pittsburgh: Harmarville Rehabilitation Center, 1972.

Malick, M. H. *Manual on Dynamic Hand Splinting with Thermoplastic Materials.* Pittsburgh: Harmarville Rehabilitation Center, 1974.

Malick, M. H. Upper Extremity Orthotics. In H. L. Hopkins and H. D. Smith (Eds.), *Willard and Spackman's Occupational Therapy* (5th ed.). Philadelphia: J.B. Lippincott, 1978.

VonPrince, K. M. P., and Yeakel, M. H. *The Splinting of Burn Patients.* Springfield, Ill.: Charles C. Thomas, 1974.

Index

Abductor digiti minimi, 5, 6
Ace bandage, as strapping material, 132
Adductor pollicis, 4, 5, 6
Adherence, of plastic splint materials, 105–107
Anatomy
 bone structure, 2–3
 musculature, 4–7
 sensory innervation, 8. *See also* Function
Angles of obliquity, 13
 in splint, 15
 and transverse metacarpal arch, 14
Antideformity position, 22
Appearance, classic
 of arthritic hand, 22
 burned hand, 22
 radial nerve severance, 20
Aquapan, 104
Aquaplast, characteristics of, 107
Arches
 carpal, 12
 longitudinal, 12
 proximal transverse, 12
 transverse metacarpal, 11
Arthritic hand, classic appearance of, 22

Bandage, plaster, 99
Bars, 30
 C, 30
 connector, 37
 cross, 35
 deviation, 34
 dorsal interosseous, 38, 39
 dorsal metacarpal, 34
 forearm, 30
 hypothenar, 32
 lumbrical, 33
 opponens, 31
 reinforcement, 35
 stabilization, 35
 wrist extensor, 29. *See also specific bars*
Bar-type long opponens splint
 construction, 88–89
 purpose of, 87
Bar-type short opponens splint
 construction, 82–87
 purpose of, 81
Bending, of splint material, 112
Bioplastic B and BX, characteristics of, 106
Bony joints, relationship of hand crease to, 9, 10
Buckle closure, 133
Burned hand, classic appearance of, 22

Carpal arch, 12
Carpalmetacarpal joint, 3
Carpal tunnel, 12
C bar
 attaching, 62
 checking for fit, 63
 with connector bar, 65, 66

determining length of, 61
determining width, 61
purpose of, 60
rolled, 69–73
Closures, 37
 buckle, 133
 D-ring, 127, 128
 safety pin, 133
 stud, 133
 types of, 127, 133
 Velcro, 127
Cloth, as strapping material, 132
Cock-up splint, 25
 with **C** bar attachment, 60
 with **C** bar and opponens attachment, 63
 with incorrectly attached ulnar
  deviation bar, 59
 palmar portion of, 54
 pattern design for, 53–56
 points of pressure in, 26
 with rolled **C** bar, 69–73
 with ulnar deviation bar, 57, 58
 wrist area in, 56
Connector bars, 37
 with **C** bar, 65, 66
 with opponens bar, 68
 purpose of, 63
Construction of splint
 bending in, 112
 curving contour, 111
 holes drilled, 114, 117
 smooth edges, 111
 stable joint, 115
 U-shaped notches in, 113
Contour curving, 111
Corners, rounding of, 68, 72, 77
Creases, hand
 marked for splinting, 49–51
 relationship to bony joints, 9
Cross bar, 35
Cylindrical grasp, 18

Design, splint, 43. *See also* Pattern
 design
Deviation bar, 34
Digits. *See* Fingers
Distal interphalangeal (DIP) joint, 3
Dorsal aspect, sensory innervation
 of, 8
Dorsal interossei, 4, 5, 6
Dorsal interosseous bar, 38, 39
Dorsal metacarpal bar, 34
Dorsal splints, 27, 80
Dorsal surface, 2
Drawing devices, for fashioning splint,
 105–107
Dressings, as strapping material, 132
D-ring, for closure, 127, 128
Dynamic assist, 38
Dynamic extension assist, 38

Edema, problem of, 3
Elastic, as strapping material, 132
Elastic memory, of splint materials,
 103–104